HOLISTIC HEALING

12 real life accounts of healing mind, body and soul by overcoming stress and burnout, processing trauma, rewiring the brain, reprogramming the mind, and integrating the soul

**Created and Compiled
by Andrea Pennington, MD, C.Ac.**

Featuring stories by:

Karan Joy Almond — Simone Anliker

Charlotte Banff — Karin Eke

Cynthia J Harrison — Siv Harstad

Kati Liebskind — Margo Livingston, PhD

Vidya Mahabaleswar — Judith Pennington

Delia Sanchez — Shelley Thomas, JD

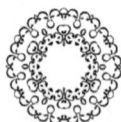

MAKE YOUR MARK GLOBAL

Holistic Healing © 2020 Andrea Pennington, Karan Joy Almond, Simone Anliker, Charlotte Banff, Karin Eke, Cynthia J Harrison, Siv Harstad, Kati Liebskind, Margo Livingston, Vidya Mahabaleswar, Judith Pennington, Delia Sanchez, Shelley Thomas

Published by Make Your Mark Global Publishing, LTD

Book cover design: Andrea Danon & Stefan Komljenović of Art Biro Network www.artbiro.ba

Library of Congress Cataloging-in-Publication Data

Library of Congress Control Number: 2020948756

Holistic Healing

Publisher: Make Your Mark Global, LTD

Las Vegas, Nevada

Pages - 154

Trade Paperback ISBN 978-1-7341526-8-5

Hardcover ISBN 978-1-7356790-0-6

Ebook ISBN 978-1-7341526-9-2

Subjects: Health, Psychology

Summary: In Holistic Healing Dr. Andrea Pennington presents 12 real life accounts of healing mind, body and soul by overcoming stress and burnout, processing trauma, rewiring the brain, reprogramming the mind, and integrating the soul. The stories include a range of conditions; breast cancer, autoimmune disease, multiple sclerosis, sciatica, depression and grief. And what these stories all have in common is how they prove that beyond the Western medical model are healing modalities that can bring new life and possibility to us to help us thrive after trauma, and experience more growth than we thought possible. There is great hope and inspiration to be found here.

MAKE YOUR MARK GLOBAL PUBLISHING, LTD

USA

For information on bulk purchase orders of this book or to book Dr. Andrea to speak at your event or on your program, call +33 06 12 74 77 09 or send an email to Booking@AndreaPennington.com

Also Compiled or Co-authored by Andrea Pennington

Manifesting Love

The Top 10 Traits of Highly Resilient People

Magic and Miracles

Life After Trauma

Time to Rise

Turning Points / Vendepunkter

Heart to Heart: The Path to Wellness

Resilience Through Yoga and Meditation

Dedication

This book is lovingly dedicated to all of the beautiful souls
who are striving to reclaim health and vitality

May this book provide you with new insights on how healing can
come in surprising ways

May you find inspiration and hope
to uncover the holistic source of true healing

Contents

Preface

The book you hold in your hands is a collection of very generous, honest stories from courageous authors. Each of them has opened up their heart to bring you insight into what led them out of pain, confusion and breakdowns into their present lives which are full of beauty, joy and light. These stories of resilience demonstrate that we are stronger than we know!

Because our authors are from a variety of countries and we are publishing these stories in English you may notice that the spelling of words is sometimes in British English and sometimes in American English, depending on the author's country of origin. You'll also see that some phrases they use are unknown to you, as they are not always direct translations from their mother tongue.

In light of the fact that many of our authors are not native English speakers, our team of editors has worked hard to make each story clear and full of the impact the author intended. It is our sincere hope that we have done their compelling stories justice and that you will be moved and inspired by them.

If you'd like to hear the authors in their own voice and watch as they provide context and color to how they decided that this is the time to break their silence I invite you to visit www.MakeYourMarkGlobal.com to watch interviews conducted by the book's publisher, Dr. Andrea Pennington.

Introduction

I was first inspired to write a book about holistic healing while talking to other medical doctors who, like myself, have since expanded their practice of medicine to include complementary and holistic treatments. Branching off into fields such as functional medicine, age management, nutrition, Traditional Chinese Medicine, Ayurveda along with mindfulness and meditation has allowed us to provide more comprehensive and effective treatment to our patients. This approach has only become mainstream in the West and incorporated into medical training in the last decade or so. Fortunately, modern science is now showing us that various approaches to comprehensive care, where we focus on treating the whole person as well as the environment, have been maintaining the health of people for thousands of years.

I first learned the holistic approach to healthcare by watching my mother, who began her career in healthcare as a nurse in England. Known today by many as Dr. P, my mother continued her education to become a doctor, and then trained further in acupuncture in the United States. As a child I followed her around the hospital when possible as she did her medical rounds. I watched her interact with patients and hospital staff with compassion and respect. She never looked at her patients as a disease, nor did she just look at the numbers on their charts. She dug deep into their minds, hearts and lives to understand the underpinnings of their illness. She provided coaching and motivation to empower them to return to health.

Surprisingly, unlike many of her contemporaries at the time, she was not quick to give out prescriptions to treat illness. She would first give patients the opportunity to fix the underlying cause of their diseases with lifestyle, nutrition, and mindset and behavior modification, always encouraging them that they had the power to heal. She had incredible faith that the human body's innate vitality code could switch on healing processes.

For example when I overheard our neighbor confide in my mother that she was feeling depressed and wondered if an antidepressant would be helpful, Dr. P asked her a series of questions that at first seemed unrelated. She asked about the woman's passions, dreams and self-care regimen. The woman replied that she had no time for herself and that she gave up on her dreams when her son was born as she just didn't have the energy for anything beyond caring for him and her husband.

My mother prodded her to return to some of the pastimes that she once enjoyed including swimming, and encouraged her to reinstitute date nights with her husband. While these interventions were simple and obvious to many of us today, for this woman they were revolutionary. The time it took her to overcome guilt for looking after her own needs and reluctance to indulge in 'me time' was time well spent. In a matter of weeks she was thanking my mom for giving her life back. She didn't need the antidepressant that many other doctors would have reflexively offered her at the time.

Of course these interventions aren't amazingly novel, but the thought process and investigation behind them are. Rather than treating a symptom with a pill, we are all being invited to look at our pain and problems to get to the root causes. Often times our body is simply showing us areas of our lives that we have ignored or hidden from ourselves. And when we explore deeply our past and present, we often find clues to our healing. And sometimes that healing is best stimulated with nonconventional therapies.

Introduction

While I was still in medical school my mother received training in acupuncture for drug and alcohol detox. She told me about how the placement of 5 tiny needles on the ear, the NADA protocol, could calm the body, brain and mind enough to help people participate in their talk therapy and 12-step meetings with decreased emotional resistance.

She soon took on a project to help pregnant women who were addicted to crack cocaine. She helped them detox from cocaine as part of an outpatient treatment program. When she told me about it I was astounded. "You can't do that", I said, worried for the patients going through withdrawal with no IV support to take the edge off the uncomfortable symptoms and shakes. In fact, having just been through a hospital rotation in psychiatry where I saw people in withdrawal from cocaine and opioids, I thought that her approach would be inhumane. Yet, there were programs being launched in various states across America as part of court-mandated drug treatment. And people were not only safely withdrawing from addictive substances, they were healing childhood trauma and staying sober for years after treatment ended.

I was curious and wanted to experience acupuncture for myself. What would these tiny needles really have to offer anybody? When I sat for my first session I was amazed. With just a few acupuncture needles in my skin, I felt the most intense energy rush and emotional release. This was when I knew my mom was on to something important and that there was certainly much more to healing than my typical medical education was providing.

I returned to medical school and I campaigned for the permission to do a rotation with the pioneer in the acu-detox treatment, the late Dr. Michael Smith. The dean of the medical school agreed and I was off to the Lincoln Hospital in the Bronx, New York for a special 6-week rotation. I learned the acupuncture protocol and a bit about Chinese herbs. In short order I was helping people to detox from drug addiction too. I gave over 100 treatments and was certain that I would take my studies further.

After medical school I attended medical acupuncture training at the Helms Institute of UCLA. I added acupuncture into each and every treatment plan I gave at the wellness institute I founded with my mother. For years we offered a mixture or eastern and western medicine, using a bio-psycho-social approach to diagnosis and treatment. I felt that I was making a genuine difference in the lives of my patients.

Having started my medical career with an open mind, I was inspired to investigate so many other treatment modalities and complimentary therapies that I can't name them all. I invited specialists to my wellness center who provided craniosacral therapy, somatic experiencing, EMDR, hypnotherapy, Traditional Chinese Medicine, nutritional detox, and breath work to name a few.

In 2000 I entered into the field of medical journalism as the Medical Director and Spokesperson for the Discovery Health Channel, which has since become the Oprah Winfrey Network. My position granted me the opportunity to be an expert guest on shows like The Oprah Winfrey Show, The Dr. Oz Show, and The Today Show multiple times, to talk about the wider picture of health. My daily presence in the media allowed my circle of influence to grow and expand which put me in contact with some of the most dynamic, pioneering healthcare providers.

Over the course of my 20+ year career I've seen that the ways that we can heal from disease, illness and trauma are so vast and numerous. This book will provide you with a sample of approaches to healing physical and emotional dis-ease and improving overall wellbeing. You will see that the holistic approach to healing involves more than looking at a disease process or the organs involved. In holistic health care we look at the whole person — mind, body and soul — as well as how they exist in their environment and relationships. We look at their thoughts, beliefs, past experiences, nutrition and movement.

The holistic approach is the opposite of our band-aid mentality that focuses on treating symptoms instead of eliminating the cause of illness. In fact, it is so incredibly rare for people to stop, step back and gain a great enough perspective on their lives to realize the actual root of the problem so they spend a lifetime medicating.

How many people who are overweight and binge eating, ever address the emotional issues which underpin their overeating? How many alcoholics heal their childhood trauma before their liver becomes diseased? How many burnt out, exhausted and depressed people press on, working in the same role that burnt them out, never understanding the psychological pattern that keeps them stuck where they are?

Most people never see the big picture, and this is perhaps one of our greatest problems today. We are all so tired, medicated to the point of numbness, and distracted that we never step off the conveyor belt to sit with our discomfort and heal it. Our life path feels automated, and from birth to death we move on autopilot.

But what if we hit the emergency stop button?

All conveyor belts do have an emergency stop button — you just have to look up to see it. The authors in this book have all found their emergency stop button through one means or another. You can either choose to look up and use it, or you fall flat on your back and find yourself finally looking up to see how you could have avoided the breakdown you're in.

When you do see it, this can just come as a sudden flash of insight at first. It can be fleeting, so you have to be willing to pay attention. But when you do finally realize that you've been on autopilot this whole time, you begin to ask yourself the questions.

How did my health get so bad?

Why am I here?

When did it all begin to go wrong and why?

As you will hear from the authors in this book, our health problems do not exist in a vacuum. A symptom or condition is the end result of your body crying out for healing when your mind would not listen.

Chronic illness really does seem like the last chance for you to pay attention to yourself. And I hope to demonstrate with this book that taking a holistic, whole view of your health incorporating body, mind and soul can heal you more deeply and completely than merely treating individual symptoms alone.

Epigenetics, Nature, Nurture, and the Body-Mind Connection

Most of us reading this book will have parents or grandparents who witnessed World War Two. Those brave souls survived through a period of human history that is traumatizing to read about, never mind experiencing it first hand.

If you delve deeper into the world of holistic health you will at some point hear about generational trauma and epigenetics. Epigenetics is the study of changes in gene expression due to external influences. In other words, this is where nature meets nurture.

Introduction

The genes we are born with are our nature. The external influences, such as traumatic events in childhood, the way we were raised, and our physical environment all contribute to how we are nurtured.

When we talk about generational trauma, there is psychological research focused on the nurturing we experienced from our caregivers. If they had complex PTSD, or at least carry some fear in back of their minds, as growing, impressionable children, we may pick up and embody some of these fears and beliefs for ourselves.

Evidence of this was famously reported in Canada in 1966, with the children of Holocaust survivors. Psychologists began to observe large numbers of these children seeking mental health services. Referrals to psychiatry clinics showed a 300% overrepresentation when it came to the children of holocaust survivors compared to the rest of the population. This is an unmissable example of trauma being handed down the generational line.

As an Integrative Physician, I have studied longitudinal studies showing that many of these children of holocaust survivors also experienced chronic physical conditions. The effects of trauma on our DNA, our mindset and coping strategies is now well understood. If you're not into reading medical studies, I do hope that as you read this book you will gain a deeper understanding of the link between mind and body.

There is a huge amount of stigma for conditions that are deemed 'psychosomatic' or that are 'all in your head,' and I have a bone to pick with that. The body-mind connection is something I feel more doctors should give real weight to when diagnosing their patients. We cannot separate the mind from the body, and indeed if we are taught in medical science that the brain is the organ impacting the health of the mind, and the brain is very much a part of our physical body, then why the stigma and why the separation?

I strongly believe that we all need to start treating the person as a whole, and not breaking patients down into groups of symptoms, or different bodily systems kept separate from the mind. Surely, humans as a species are intelligent enough to recognize that we are more than the sum of our physical parts.

As we move through the sections of this book together, I hope that my contributing authors and I can arm you with sufficient knowledge and inspiration that you begin seeing yourself as all that you are — a magnificent and complex being — and not just flesh, bone and symptoms.

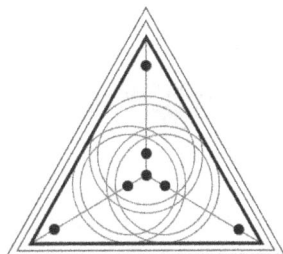

Part 1
Self Belief and the
Narrative of Healing

It has been said that if you expect to see good things, then you will. But of course, it is also true that the more you expect to experience the bad things in life, the more negativity and suffering will come your way.

"The Law of Attraction states that whatever you focus on, think about, read about, and talk about intensely, you're going to attract more of into your life."

~ Jack Canfield

We have long been able to draw a line of correlation between people who have a difficult start in life to those who experience chronic illness later down the track. As a physician with a special interest in trauma and resilience, this is an issue very close to my heart. Early in my career I realized that people who had an internal belief that they were bad, flawed, or undeserving of love and happiness didn't heal as well as those who believed they were worthy of love and inherently good.

Throughout this book I will refer to many common themes in the world of healing holistically; from our belief systems to manifestation, and to the importance of the narrative we each have for ourselves. In this section we will particularly focus on the role of narrative, that is the story we tell ourselves about ourselves. We will explore how personal narrative impacts the path of becoming unwell, and how it influences healing.

We will also return often to the topic of Adverse Childhood Experiences (ACEs), as this will shed a great deal of light on the correlation between childhood stress and chronic illness. The tricky thing about the adversity we experience in childhood is that it sets the tone for the adult life we will grow into. As children, we naturally accept the world around us. If we are abused or neglected, we absorb the belief that we deserved that fate. This in turn typically grows into a poor relationship with ourself, lacking in self-love and abundant in toxic stress. So it's not hard to see why the correlation between childhood stress and adult illness is so common. But the really good news is that this can be changed for the better.

"You manifest what you believe, not what you want."

~ Sonia Ricotti

The narrative that runs in our mind and informs our life choices has much to do with this. When we are stuck in our childhood narrative of victimhood, the lack of love for ourself manifests in myriad unhealthy behaviors. From perfectionism and overwork, to a lack of physical care for ourselves, we can soon end up burnt out and sick.

When we constantly tell ourselves that we will become ill, or when we fear illness, we are focused on it. This becomes the outcome that we manifest. Working on that narrative and learning to love ourselves for the brave, resilient survivors we are, then gives way to decreased stress, a calmer nervous system, less inflammation and disease. The list of benefits is nearly endless.

You may have read Dying To Be Me by Anita Moorjani, it's a very famous book. Many people have picked up a copy, primarily interested in the NDE (near death experience) Anita had when her cancer had spread throughout her body. But the really big message Anita had for us is different. Rather than focusing on the fact that she left her body and came back to this world, the resounding message or moral of the story is about what caused her cancer.

Where her NDE gave her some profound insights into the meaning of life, she came back to Earth with the understanding that her fear of cancer had been the reasons she manifested it in her own body. She was so fearful and stressed by seeing her friend die of cancer, and had focused so much on restricting her diet and, in essence, restricting her enjoyment of life, that she had thought cancer into her world.

Both in my early medical career, and in my more recent years as a publisher, I've met so many people who have shown me the power of our beliefs and our inner dialogue. We cannot separate the mental from the physical, and we truly can think things into our reality. The stories in this first section demonstrate how, for these authors, their initial lack of love for themselves, or expectation that they would suffer, lead them to become ill.

You will hear from Kati, Karan Joy, and Margo, three women who tried a range of medical and complementary interventions for their illnesses, but ultimately needed to reconnect with themselves and focus on their mind and spirit just as much, if not more, than their physical ailments. Focusing on more positive outcomes, and on more positive stories for themselves gave them the shift they needed to turn their health around.

How Intuition Healed Me from Breast Cancer

by Kati Liebeskind

Imagine how you would feel if someone told you your life could be over soon. I had this experience when I was very young, as a university student about to graduate. I studied psychology and English in the USA, Oregon and Miami to be exact. I was a good student and loved travelling and adventures. When I lived in Miami, I got to swim with a dolphin.

I wrote my research paper for my master's degree about cognitive learning processes. Therefore I did empirical research in a bilingual school in Seattle. After my exciting experiences in the US, I enrolled for my final written and oral exams in Germany. I studied for my exams in my beautiful apartment located in the forest in Kassel where I always felt like I was on vacation.

My life was never boring. I had 3 jobs, worked on weight training and studied for my final exams. I was full of energy and excited for all the possibilities after my graduation. I still had my whole life ahead of me.

In the summer of 2005 everything changed. I began to feel very tired. I had too much on my plate. I worried sometimes about who would take care of me if I got sick. Then, I went to my gynaecologist. I did not expect things could get worse. She did an ultrasound of my breasts and informed me: "Something doesn't look good in your right breast." She transferred me to a specialist for a biopsy.

First I thought: "It won't be anything serious."

A few days after the biopsy the doctor sent the diagnosis to my gynaecologist. "You need to see me. It's urgent", she said. I went to her, knowing deep down something was out of alignment with my health.

When she said: "It's cancer." I could not say a word. My body was frozen like an ice block. She continued, her words overwhelming me. "It is urgent. You need surgery. I recommend two hospitals."

I said the only thing I could in that moment: "Please give me some time to think about it." I left the doctor's office and crossed the marketplace. It was noisy there, but I only heard the noise in my head. "What should I do? I don't know what I can do? I have to choose a doctor. Which doctor should I choose?" Questions flooded my brain.

Finally, the noise in my head stopped. I was crying. Suddenly someone patted me on the shoulder. I turned back and saw my girlfriend that I had not seen in years. She asked: "Why are you crying?"

I said: "I came from my gynaecologist. She found something in my breast." My girlfriend immediately hugged me. Then she said one of her friends had gone through the same thing recently. She gave me her friend's number and I called her. She explained how happy she was that she went to the right clinic for treatment. "The head doctor is a specialist for breast-reconstruction. He even worked in the USA."

When I heard the word "USA" I knew where I needed to go. This answer felt good in my body. I loved the USA. But my intuition was also overshadowed with doubt and a lot of fear. I was a head person. I did not show my feelings, even though being an empath and highly sensitive are my natural talents.

A week passed and I had another appointment with my gynaecologist. She asked:: "Did you decide which hospital you would like to choose?" The fear welled up inside of me and I was still unsure, even though my body and my intuition gave me a clear sign of what I needed to do.

My doctor said: "You need to trust." Suddenly, I went out of my head into my feelings and intuition and found myself saying: "I will see the doctor who worked in the USA."

After I got the diagnosis, I was in shock. I could not think clearly. I was just functioning because I had to. I decided to have the surgery and I prayed from the bottom of my heart that I wouldn't lose my breast.

After the surgery, I still had my breast but the doctor explained he would discuss my case with other doctors if chemotherapy was necessary. It took 7 days. This was the longest week of my entire life. I prayed that I would not lose my long hair if chemo was needed. All of my prayers were heard.

I still had my breast, a little bit smaller with a small scar that was barely visible. I did not get chemo. But the doctors said it was necessary to do radiation and take pills that put me in menopause.

When I got out of the hospital, a lot of family stuff came up for me. Nobody in my family could show their feelings about the situation. My brother, whom I really love, visited me just once in the hospital, which made me think nobody would truly care if I died. This helped me make my next big decision – I wasn't going to get any further treatments. I was ok with the idea of dying, but I wanted to experience love first.

I did not fight anymore against the cancer. I surrendered and I cried. I cried a lot. All the pressure came out of me. It was a release. I let all of my feelings bubble up, like soap bubbles, until they popped and dissipated. Finally, I felt at peace. Some ideas came to me. I felt I needed a psychologist. I saw three different psychologists but could not find one who resonated with me.

I decided to do the radiation and hormone therapy. The pills made me very tired. I started to sweat a lot because I was in menopause. It was a hard experience to go through at such a young age. The clinic where I did the radiation had a social worker. And the doctor told me if I was interested in getting a spa treatment to go see the social worker. All patients in Germany have access to a spa treatment that is covered by insurance after a major illness. Patients with public health insurance can stay in clinics for public patients. Patients who have private health insurance can stay in private clinics. I was covered by public health insurance.

From that point on everything changed in my life. I learned a lot about the right holistic healing methods for my body. I followed my intuition. Miracles happened in surprising ways.

The social worker in the radiation clinic gave me brochures about public spa clinics for cancer patients. I did not know which spa clinic would be good for me. Then out of the blue an idea came to me. I remembered when I was hiking in Kassel, I saw a beautiful private clinic called Habichtswaldklinik. Once I went inside and was fascinated by the beautiful interior.

I liked the white couches, the beautiful carpets red and gold in an Indian design and the big colourful mandala pictures on the walls in the lobby. I thought: "One day, when I earn good money, I will come here." I remembered how I felt there and I said with a very small voice to the social worker: "I like the Habichtswaldklinik in Kassel, but it is a private clinic." The social worker said: "Well, we will just have to give it a try."

She filled out the forms for the spa application and sent it to my retirement insurance. They made a mistake. Therefore, the retirement insurance sent the form to my health insurance. My health insurance said: "The retirement insurance needs to pay for you." Then the retirement insurance realized their mistake and said to my health insurance. "We will cover all of the expenses." Then the health insurance said to me: "When your retirement insurance pays for everything, we will allow you to stay in the Habichtswaldklinik." I was so happy I would be able to stay in this wonderful private clinic for 5 weeks.

I felt like a princess. They had Ayurvedic cuisine and Ayurvedic massages. The air was filled with the fragrance of massage oils. In Ayurveda they have three Doshas according to a person's body structure and personality, Vata, Ptta and Kapha. The Ayurvedic cuisine offers different meals for each Dosha, sweet, spicy and sharp. They use different massage oils that smell different for each individual type. I learned about orthomolecular supplements and meditation. This clinic is directly connected with the Kurhessen Therme. Each day, I could go through a long tunnel to a big indoor spa with salt water hot springs, water fountains and saunas.

A very good psychotherapist worked there. His clients came from Hamburg and drove four hours in order to see him. There were also other psychologists employed in the Habichtswaldklinik. I wanted the best one. I could not go to him because he was overbooked. One lady who went to him suggested putting a note in his mailbox. So I did.

He called me for an appointment. When I went to him he said he was overbooked, but asked where I lived. When I told him Kassel he asked: "Do you have private insurance? If you do I could offer you some appointments after your spa." I told him I only had public health insurance and that I was a student. The psychotherapist told me that a rich lady who died gave all of her money to the Habichtswaldklinik in a foundation. "This foundation is there for people in need. You could fill out a form and try to get some money." I got a scholarship so I was able to see the psychotherapist that I wanted each week.

When I had the breast surgery, they cut out some lymph nodes to check if there were metastatic tumours. Therefore, I had a lot of pain and could not lift up my right arm. I tried a couple physical therapists, but they could not help me. I met a woman with back pain at the Habichtswaldklinik and I wished her a good recovery. She told me, out of the blue, that she went to an osteopath outside of the Habichtswaldklinik. I told her about the pain I had when I moved my right arm. She replied: "Perhaps you could try this osteopath. He is the best. He is always overbooked, but I will give you his phone number."

I called him right away. His assistant said: "A lady cancelled her appointment. You can have her appointment in one hour if you have time." I went to him and learned a lot about osteopathy. It was really helpful for my arm. I had so much luck. My psychotherapist called me "Lucky mushroom." But I know now it was not luck.

I know that everything is energy. Our brain has frequencies. I realized when I thought and felt in positive ways, loving, joyful and trustful emotions, I attracted positive outcomes. When I had negative emotions like fear, worry and doubt, I manifested negative situations and health regressions.

After the spa I learned techniques to release old and unhealthy emotions. These spiritual seminars changed the way I lived my life. I let go of a lot of negative emotions that I stored inside of my body, emotions that affected my health in a negative way. After a while, I had more confidence about natural healing methods. I did a lot for my body on my own. I trained my arm twice a week. My body needed warm food, so I ate a warm meal two times a day. I trusted the signals of my body. I went grocery shopping each day and followed my natural impulses regarding what my body needed to eat that day. I took minerals and vitamins to strengthen my immune system. I learned a lot and applied what I learned to my daily life.

But I still felt tired. I knew I needed to throw away the hormone pills I'd been taking. But I was also unsure if they were keeping the cancer at bay. Finally I said bravely to my doctor: "I will not take these pills anymore." She encouraged my decision. "Trust your feelings"; she said. "You need to stand 100% behind your decision." At that moment, I trusted my body and my intuition. I also finished my master's degree with good grades.

In 2015 they did a cat scan on my breasts, just as a preventive measure. They found something abnormal in my left breast. A lot of fear came up again. But this time, I did not doubt that my thoughts and emotions could heal my left breast. I needed to do more spiritual work in order to increase my energy.

I discovered the healing power of sound and music and how it was balm to my wounded spirit. I felt all of my emotions as they came up. I also continued to eat healthy and took supplements. After six months I went to the clinic for another cat scan and the doctor did not see anything that looked like cancer. That's when I knew I could heal myself. I believed that it was possible. I believed in the healing power of love. I believed that I would always be supported by a higher force, from God.

Lessons from my journey

During my long journey to health, I discovered that it is essential to take care of my physical, mental, emotional and spiritual wellbeing in order to feel well and healthy. I learned to ask people for help who offered me the just what I needed at the right time. It was important to overcome my fear of being sick and of dying. I needed to express all of my emotions because they are a part of me. And I needed to stand up for myself and my needs and wishes. When I stood up for myself and had the belief that anything was possible, when I did not doubt myself, then miracles happened for me. The impossible became possible.

All of my experiences showed me that I have all the power that I need inside of myself, a healing power that is greater than my doubts and fears. I learned that being brave always leads to miraculous outcomes and rewards. I learned that a higher force, I call it God, is always there to lead me on my path. I just need to follow my intuition. I found the root cause of my sickness. I found love, unconditional love in myself, that is capable of healing everything.

I am cancer free since that traumatic experience. I healed myself and I continued to love my life, my body, my intuition and my sensitivity.

We are all here on this planet to be healthy and happy. It is our birthright. We are here to share the diamond that we are with the world. When we treat our physical, mental, emotional and spiritual body like a valuable diamond, we can shine healthy, happy, fulfilled while sharing our light in the world.

I would like to inspire and empower you to trust your intuition, Be brave. And treat your body like a diamond.

About the Author

I am passionate about holistic health methods and work as a psychologist, helping my clients holistically to overcome their fears and limiting beliefs. I invented a program that is new to the German market that involves fear releasing techniques combined with swimming classes and aqua training. It is easier to release fears and trauma in the water where I often work with my clients.

I built a company based on this program and took part in a Chamber of Commerce and Industry competition where I competed against 66 other companies. I received the 5th place for the most innovative company. My 8-step coaching program outside of the water has helped clients improve their health through holistic healing as well as find love and even unexpected blessings of money.

Currently I am fulfilling my dearest heart's desire to become a doctor in Natural Medicine and Quantum Healing. My heart is full of gratitude and happiness because this has been my dream since I was 14 years old.

You can find me at:
http://agape-liebeskind.de
https://m.facebook.com/kati.liebeskind
https://linkedin.com/in/kati-liebeskind-30b269115

Healing the Narrative, Wholistically

by Karan Joy Almond

I always knew I was on a journey to find or do something profound. Rivaling a search for the Holy Grail, I would go into every nook and cranny of experience hoping to find the answer. Over time, I became brave and would pull a Kathy Bates from her scene in Fried Green Tomatoes. "TOWANDA," and damn the consequences. I would soon learn that profound comes in fascinating ways!

I would like to say I was born courageous but that would be a lie. I was born knowing that I did not belong here, that I was missing some mysterious piece of the puzzle of ME! By the time I would develop the courage to go "TOWANDA" on life, I would have experienced multiple traumas that would, literally change my personality in ways that no one could see ME. They only saw the great wall of protection I had built. This happened organically over time. I felt desperate to be connected to another human being that I could trust. Yet, time after time, I would put my trust in people who would betray me. Betrayal was my nemesis, and then through extraordinary loss, it became the teacher that would finally bring me back into my body, mind, and Spirit.

I will return to that point, but first, I would like to set the stage to help you understand that I am in no way unique or different than any other human who has experienced and tried to process the type of traumatic life events for which we have no instruction manual. Trauma, for some, can be momentary and released as quickly as it occurs. For others, we allow it to permeate our cellular memory like a black ink that oozes into our veins, turning all the color and beauty available to us into a heavy, muddy mess. Most of us, especially empaths, have no real awareness as this occurs. We experience a subsequent event, often referred to as a "trigger," that causes an immediate release of the biochemical hiccup that happened with the original trauma.

This is a very deep topic that cannot be fully explained here, but this is the core truth that I had to understand before I could heal my body, mind, and Spirit.

My mind (emotions) had been sick for a very long time. My early years were confusing and painful. While my parents loved me without condition and provided for me, I came to realize that my parents had their own personal traumas and that their precious newborn also came without an instruction manual. My bottom line here is that parental blame is useless and only keeps the narrative of familial trauma alive.

My Spirit was an interesting study for me. Around the age of 35, the concept of "calling your Spirit back" was presented to me. What I would come to understand is there is no real mystery or magic to that process if we learn to live our authentic truths rather than the "conditioning" of familial, cultural, societal, religious, and political influence. These external factors block our ability to have our internal and external selves remain congruent.

I believe that this is where real illness begins.

I had been unable to listen to Spirit on my own behalf until my body and mind became so broken that I had to realize resistance was presenting an exhaustive repetitive cycle. I had to admit that I knew nothing, and that I was ready to do whatever would be asked of me to find my way back to being whole again. Much was asked and I admit there were moments that I cursed that agreement, but I always came back to my desire to heal.

For me, a long circuitous path down the rabbit hole of acute injury and disabling chronic illness would be the final call from Spirit for me to stop fighting and listen. On my birthday, January 2, 2018, at 3:33 am, I was in a lucid dream state and heard the words, "standing in the shadow of my own light." That lucid dream state, similar to a life review, ended with me being fully awake and crying tears of regret and joy. I realized that my loss of vitality and zest for life had simply been about living an incongruent life in which I was screaming one thing on the inside but often outwardly expressing the opposite.

My resistance to Spirit had been my own delusional perception that my own Spirit had deceived me by allowing me to be in a position of betrayal by others; by life. By now, I think you are aware that my Achilles' heel had been betrayal after betrayal. While I could write a book about those life experiences, I have also come to understand that I had to let go of that narrative to make room for a new narrative about life as I desired it to be. Suffice it to say, that my real "come to Jesus" moment was when I admitted that I put myself in the position to be betrayed. My Spirit had attempted to give me warning after warning, but I had been so traumatized that I continued to seek evidence and attempt to figure out the future before I allowed a decision to be made.

Therefore, life happened *to* me rather than *for* me.

You might be wondering what this has to do with the topic of this book, Holistic Healing. As I said, my final call came in the form of an illness that would become neurologically disabling and lead doctors to predict I would not recover. Four-and-a- half years of multiple-antibiotic therapy and narcotics left me so depleted that I remained in bed, in a dark room for the better part of 12 years.

I described my "call to action" in the book, *Time To Rise,* in which I manifested an acceptable diagnosis, cancer, as a way to just leave this planet and get a do-over. I now see clearly how Spirit worked on my behalf in a way that now seems hilarious to me. But first, I had to feel the anger that I had kept contained; until the brain inflammation no longer allowed me to process incoming information and parse it out rationally. The rages were temporary but powerful, and they scarred my ex-husband and children in ways I would prefer not to admit to. However regretful I feel, I now understand that Spirit allows everyone the experience they need to grow, and sometimes those experiences are not so pleasant. Childbirth is not all that pleasant either, but the potential for the greatest gift of life at the end allows mothers to accept the pain.

Just as I began to recover some of my function in 2011, I would get the final hit that would force me to change the trajectory of my life in ways that would bring me the exact desires I had journaled about for many years, but had believed were unattainable. I was cured from melanoma. Yes, that was my call to action but I still was not willing to let the narrative of illness go and allow Spirit to direct me. In typical Capricorn fashion, I went about trying every holistic, integrative, and functional medical approach and any off-the-grid treatment, therapy, or gadget I could find. Some of the "healthy" diet options I tried (namely experimenting with raw food), ended up being a mistake for me. I was still using my mind to try and force my body to heal. That caused some nutritional and gut issues that led me to discover the dangers of mercury amalgam fillings. True to my nature, I jumped in and immediately used my mind to make a choice where Spirit must have held a meeting and asked, "What the actual fuck ARE we going to have to do to her?"

Once I read about the dangers of amalgam fillings, I saw a dentist who would remove one of them but it was without protection from the mercury vapor that is released with the slightest friction. Unfortunately, my compromised immune system and structural tooth damage would require a decision to either undergo a root canal or extract the tooth. I was referred to a biological dentist, who eventually saved my life, figuratively and probably literally. However, for several reasons, I chose to go to an endodontist first and try to save my teeth.

Over the next eighteen months, I ended up having root canals in my entire upper right quadrant and all lower molars. This means the blood supply was severed and the three miles of microtubules that surround the filled root make nice little condominiums for anaerobic organisms to hang out and litter the immune system with their noxious excrement.

I would suffer to the point that the endodontist moved me on to the chief pain management dentist at the University of Maryland Dental School, and I was left wearing a prosthetic cup that I had to fill with ketamine, a tranquilizer, every hour to tolerate the neuropathic pain in my mouth, jaw, and face. Ultimately, I would lose eleven teeth and endure thirty-one dental surgeries. Still, I would not change that for anything. It catapulted me toward the happiness I longed for.

I could also write a single book on that experience, but the point I wish to make is that, just like I did with my healthcare choice, I initially sought what I thought was safe rather than take the risk with a more holistic approach. In the end, I came to some realizations and these are the messages I want to leave you with in this chapter.

There is a big difference between acute and chronic illness. Medical academia is geared toward acute care, in which pharmaceuticals and surgeries are seen to be more efficient and effective than using the basic building blocks of our biology: vitamins, minerals, fats, amino acids, and herbs which have multiple constituents that work synergistically. Pharmaceutical companies isolate active ingredients and synthesize them in a lab. Bitter herbs are all but avoided in the SAD (Standard American Diet). Lifelong use of these building blocks will go a very long way to homeostasis and the avoidance of chronic illness. However, with a little patience and research into the process of unwinding the biological damage to the body, we can return to a state of balance, given that we are willing to understand that symptoms in the body are simply the "expression" of a bigger picture that is often missed, even in "Holistic" healthcare. Therefore, I prefer the term Wholistic.

Wholistic healthcare, to me, is the process of bringing the WHOLE of a person into balance and alignment. We have three basic parts of our being. The body (physical), the mind (emotional), and the Spirit (energetic) are part of every being, no matter your belief system, religious preference or lack thereof. My realization that living an incongruent life based on the denials, resistance, projections, and every other deflective action I took due to allowing trauma to inhabit my body, mind, and Spirit, kept me stuck in the defensive posture of survival mode — to my own detriment. The end result was a weakened vibrational state that allowed chronic illness to take root and become part of my narrative.

Narrative is a unique animal. If we want to heal ourselves wholistically, it is critical to deconstruct the story we tell ourselves when we are so busy using our mind to attempt to control external events and future outcomes. This is where we can progress by leaps and bounds if we allow Spirit to become our "therapist." The bonus is that it is free! Just let that sink in for a moment. We come with a free instruction manual and a free therapist for those times we do not listen. It is a rare external source that tells us this, so it's totally understandable that we end up fragmented and broken beings. Still Spirit is there, patiently waiting to act on our behalf.

There is one caveat to this. We have free will and are allowed to direct Spirit with our thoughts. Spirit is bound by universal law to give us what we focus on. Therefore, if we focus on what we do not want ... then guess what? That is what we will get. So, when we make our trauma, negative life experiences, and illness our story, as in "Hi, I'm Karan and I have neurological Lyme complex ..." and use that to preface and explain away our life, Spirit is getting a directive from us.

In my case, I had severe brain injury due to Lyme encephalitis and that was, legitimately, quite traumatic for someone who had always been both left- and right-brained and able to intuit things long before others were finished explaining something. In what seemed like an instant, I was unable to think my way out of a box or trust that I even understood what someone was saying to me. However, hyperbaric oxygen chamber therapy and lion's mane (mushroom) added to my Lyme treatment brought much improvement. My lack of confidence and residual cognitive issues kept me habitually "pre-explaining" my disability so others would not judge me. Therefore, I came across as dense and incapable, the very thing I wished to avoid. As an example, once I changed my narrative, and trusted Spirit to have my back as I re-entered human existence again, the word blocking and forgetfulness improved dramatically.

Therefore, I no longer wish to use my old narrative of illness to describe how truly dark of a time all that was for me. The nature of my work requires me to share some things I used to help manage symptoms while I healed, but I now prefer to tell the story of how all those external treatments, even the holistic ones, were still just bandaids for my body until I began to change my narrative and listen to Spirit. I won't pretend I just made that decision and then everything was butterflies and sunshine. It wasn't. I had to unwind the habit of fighting everything.

After dropping the narrative of illness and regaining my function, Spirit went about rearranging my life to give me exactly what I had been asking for. I had to go through a two-year period of extreme loss in my personal life, in which people who knew my story and I questioned, "just how much more can one person take?" Turns out, I am one resilient gal!

Now, here I sit writing this story in complete awe of my journey back to myself. I no longer see any of the trauma as unnecessary. It made me strong, courageous, and able to transform a negative feeling into something that feels better. I feel wholeness, joy and peace. So, to life, I now say "TOWANDA!" To Spirit, gratitude for the gift of meeting my authentic self. I now know that I do belong here. What more profound realization was there to discover on this journey?

About the Author

Karan is currently an Oral-Systemic Consultant and partners with Eric Gerson to help clients take a deeper look at past experience, beliefs, and traumas that may present in the form of unexplainable symptoms of body/mind/spirit. While unraveling these issues can take time and work, it does work over time for those who are ready and willing to take back their power as part of the healing journey.

Karen and Eric's passion is to partner with Lightworkers who are just waking up to the gifts they have to share and wish to take a more introspective and compassionate approach to their own authentic truths!

To inquire about working with Karan on dental issues relative to chronic symptoms send an email to lionsandgoats@lightworkforlightworkers.com

Or join our Holistic Dentistry support group https://www.facebook.com/groups/1491839717746119

To inquire about working with Eric and Karan to discover where you got stuck in a vibration that does not match your inner truth visit us our website lightworkforlightworkers.com or join our Facebook group: https://www.facebook.com/groups/937306003443582/

From Life-Changing Trauma to Transcendence

by Margo Livingston, PhD

"There are wounds that never show on the body that are far deeper and more hurtful than anything that bleeds."

~ Laurell K. Hamilton

Everything went pear-shaped

I was lucky enough to be born in Africa, in beautiful colonial Rhodesia (now Zimbabwe), with healthy, loving parents and a wonderful big sister, Judi. My parents were Scottish but my father, having trained the Kenyan Rifle Guards during the war, had fallen in love with Africa and had emigrated there as soon as the war was over.

I was a happy tomboy, mischievous and funny. I loved playing in our big garden with my beloved Rhodesian Ridgeback, Bruno who allowed me and Judi to scramble all over him and ride him like a horse! Mum and Dad were so proud of our home and were saving up for a long holiday over Christmas in Simonstown, near Cape Town in South Africa. I know all of this because my mum religiously wrote home to her mother and described every detail of their plans and excitement for the 2000-mile journey we would make by car in December 1963. I don't remember much about the journey or our arrival in Simonstown but I know that my parents shared the driving and my father started feeling unwell during our stop off in Johannesburg. He became increasingly unwell and lay in the back of the estate car quietly and bravely as Mum undertook most of the driving.

We arrived at the hotel "Rhodesia by the Sea" in the late afternoon. Mum ordered "sundowners", a ritual gin and tonic that they both enjoyed as the sun came down in Africa. Dad said that he felt tired and wanted to lie down. He suddenly collapsed, struggling for breath, unable to speak, gripping his head as if in agony. She called for help and knelt over Andrew, her beloved husband, in total disbelief, paralysed with fear and helplessness. My father died that night of a brain haemorrhage, aged just thirty-nine. Mum was thirty six, Judi was eight and I was just six. Mum didn't know a soul in Simonstown. How she coped, I have no idea. It was the end of her world. She had to pick herself up, whilst her heart was breaking, and be strong for Judi and me. She arranged the cremation and drove us all the way back to Salisbury (now Harare) where her mother was waiting to support her. She had come all the way from Scotland.

I didn't realise what a profound impact this event would have on my life from that moment forward. I couldn't understand where my father had gone. He hadn't said goodbye and I missed him so much. He had been the strength of the family, the decision-maker, the breadwinner, the adventurer, the fun guy at parties, the one who had dried my hair after our bath and had made me giggle. He had been strict but kind, teaching us good manners and respect for others. Mum, understandably, decided that we should return to Scotland, so she could get a job and be near her parents for support. It was soon after this time that I realised my mother was really worried about money. She had relied totally on my father for income since arriving in Africa although she was a hairdresser and they'd had an established salon back in Glasgow before moving abroad.

I didn't realise that she was planning to leave our beloved Bruno behind. We all went out in the car one day and she took us to a farm. She left Bruno there. I could not believe it – I was in the back of the car screaming as I watched him run after the car. I couldn't bear to lose him as well. How could my mother do this? She didn't even ask us. I didn't realise that even more trauma was being implanted in my subconscious. I had lost my father, my home, my country and now my dog. I was bereft.

Life as we know it – my Western upbringing and education

I grew up in Glasgow as a rebel and non-conformist. I didn't make friends easily, unlike my adorable and sensible sister. When I started school, I remember being mocked and ridiculed about my school bag being different and the "liberty bodice" that my mother forced us to wear in case we got cold. I had a different accent and the kids asked me to "speak African" and whether or not I lived in a "mud hut". I always felt remote and apart from everyone. My aunts and uncles used to say, "Smile, it can't be that bad". I wanted to be a good girl and please Mum so that she'd have less to worry about, so I studied hard at school. This became my focus – it was the only thing I could control. I excelled at school and university and graduated in 1978 as an immunologist.

I didn't know much about boys and was a bit afraid of them. I had no boyfriends until a local boy, seven years older than me, asked me out and, eventually said, "If I asked you to marry me, would you?" It wasn't exactly a romantic proposal but he was a civil engineer who was totally logical and analytical, so what did I expect? I got married at twenty-one and immediately asked Doug if we could "go to Africa". He duly acquiesced and gave up a secure job in management with British Rail to travel to Africa and work on a railway project in Algeria. I was so excited but I was soon disillusioned as when I stepped off the plane, all I saw were Arabs. I was so naïve but quickly adapted to my new adventure and loved living in the sun in a mad, crazy environment full of hustle and bustle, interesting food, smells and customs. I wanted to work and decided to return to the UK to study nursing as no one in Algeria had heard of immunology yet!

Between 1979 and 1993 I lived and worked in Algeria, Liberia, Hong Kong and had my three beloved children. I knew, however, that I was not "in love" and that my relationship was not fulfilling. I did not yet understand that I was an emotional cripple who felt that I needed a father figure to look after me financially. I did not feel deserving of true love and all the emotions this evokes.

My job in Hong Kong was so inspiring. I helped co-found the Hong Kong Marrow Match Foundation. I pioneered the DNA tissue typing techniques which helped determine bone marrow compatibility between unknown potential donors and those of Chinese origin who required a bone marrow transplant for leukaemia. I loved my job and I felt inspired by my ability to help those in need, and potentially save their lives.

My world came crashing down once again, however, when Doug's job ended and we had to leave. His job had paid for the apartment and schooling for the children so it was not an option for me to stay. I tried to work out a way but I was only paid a local salary and had to admit defeat. This was a major epiphany for me as I had had my choices removed once again. Now, I had no choice but to leave my great life in Hong Kong. I vowed that I would continue with my PhD that I'd started at Hong Kong University, no matter where. I also decided that I had to leave Doug so that I could make my own decisions from now on!

The Universe was calling me but more trauma was in store

I settled in Glasgow and completed my PhD in cancer research. I struggled as a single parent with no financial savvy. I chanced upon network marketing in the early nineties and was lured into the belief that I could become wealthy by building a network and selling health products. I see this time as a period of insanity. I was blinded by my desire to make money and scared that I could not do so "without a man". I excelled in this role, however, built several successful networks in the wellbeing industry and discovered that I was a good public speaker. I was able to inspire others with my passion and sincerity.

I have a deep desire to help people and this period introduced me to the world of personal development. I finally saw that I had been running my life on autopilot, struggling with limiting beliefs caused by a lack of self-love, lack of feeling I was enough, lack of self-worth, self-hatred, powerlessness and fear around money. I learnt that, deep down, I believed that all men would let me down and leave me because, unwittingly, that is what my father had done.

In 1995, my beloved sister Judi died of glioblastoma, an aggressive type of brain tumour. She had been a medical doctor and had four beautiful daughters, the youngest of whom was three when she died. Judi died just after her fortieth birthday. Later, I realised that Judi's illness may have come about partly because she'd bottled up her grief, always thinking of others, showing a stiff upper lip and not releasing her true emotions, unlike me.

I was bereft once again. I felt that it should have been me. Judi had been such a good person who was always doing the right thing. I was the rebel who kept getting things wrong. I felt guilty that I was alive and she was not. This shook me to the core. I realised how much my mother must be going through and how fortunate my children were to have their mother. I was depressed and sad all the time. I felt that I was emotionally unavailable to my children and not there to help them in their formative years as I was so busy soul searching.

Still seeking financial success, I turned to stock-broking as I could not get funding to continue my scientific career. I really disliked the corporate world. It seemed cutthroat and heartless, only focused on profit, with no regard for the customers' well-being. I became more stressed and unfocused in my life. I started drinking too much alcohol in the evenings, trying to block out the pain and loss I was trying to process. Suddenly, the universe stepped in and made a declaration which forced me to literally stop dead and re-evaluate my life.

I had developed cataracts in both eyes which was unusual for my age. I needed a routine operation for artificial lenses. Cataract literally means "a great downpour; a deluge". This proved to be inauspicious as my routine operation turned out to be a major disaster. During the procedure, I heard the surgeon say, "This scalpel is blunt" and "There's not enough irrigation fluid in this machine". I knew that I was doomed. Afterwards, he came and told me that most of my lens had gone into the back of my eye. It is supposed to be pulverised and sucked up by their equipment to avoid this. I developed a detached retina overnight.

The surgeon, clearly mortified by what had happened, came round to my house personally with a referral letter for the retinal team. During my second operation in two days for an emergency retinal repair, my retina detached further and my eye started to bleed internally. They told me later that they had been about to remove my eye as they had not been able to control the bleeding and had been afraid it would affect the other eye. By some miracle, the eye stopped bleeding and I was told not to expect to regain much, if any, vision, in my left eye. I was forced to lie, face down, for six weeks, in an attempt to heal as much of the retina as possible.

This was a catharsis for me as I was forced to stop my life, stop my manic running around trying to survive and be everything to everyone and accept help, love and support from my family. I lay there thinking about my life, about all the mistakes I felt I had made, about the people I felt I had let down, about my beloved children and how lost they must feel, about the agony of loss of my sister and father. I cried a lot at that time. I thought about suicide. I literally couldn't 'see' a way out. Interestingly, my employer, the stockbroker, made me redundant while I was off sick. Could it get any worse?

The transformation – when West meets East

"The natural healing force within each of us is the greatest force in getting well."

~ Hippocrates

I started listening to meditation music, seeking solace from my thoughts. I listened to inspiring recordings about people overcoming trauma and seemingly insurmountable difficulties. I began to understand that I had been given a divine gift, the gift of being forced to stop my hectic life, to re-evaluate and change to a path of spirituality. I could make my own choices based on integrity, love and compassion for myself and others. I willed myself to heal. I visualised my vision returning and imagined hugging my children, reading them stories, seeing beautiful sunsets, the beauty of spring, smelling the lovely flowers in my garden, driving again and travelling around the world. I began to see a glimmer of light – both literally and metaphorically.

I awoke one morning and saw some light coming through the curtains. I was beside myself with joy. The doctors were amazed at the vision I recovered. I cannot see well out of my left eye but I can see shapes and colours, far more than they ever expected. I promised myself that, from this point, I would live a life of spiritual connection, love and peace. I would study eastern traditions and healing modalities which would keep me healthy and continuously improve my physical and emotional healing process.

I steered away from corporate business, trained as an advanced nurse practitioner and started my own business as a health consultant. I studied Qi Gong, body sculpting and optimal nutrition, became a Feng

Shui and bioenergetics consultant and practised every day to improve my thinking and my health. Qi Gong was life-changing as it helped me focus, remain calm and centred and helped remove any aches and pains. I developed my own healing practice and worked one on one with those suffering from many ailments, including insomnia, grief, arthritis, high blood pressure and gastrointestinal issues.

I continued to have ups and downs due to more traumatic events, which led me to the proven psychotherapeutic approach which addresses our thoughts and resultant reality through the Three Principles, pioneered by Sydney Banks.

I have been tested to my limits on many occasions and now realise that resilience is within us all. Our stories help make us strong and are an example to others that it is possible to heal, that any obstacle can be overcome through love, forgiveness and self-belief. It is our thoughts about our circumstances which bring us the greatest suffering.

I am passionate about healing. I see this as a five-pillared approach to wellbeing. I realise that we mostly all have innate mental and physical health; that our body has the template for recovery, far more so than any man-made medication; and that we can only heal ourselves and others through love and forgiveness. Using a combined focus on internal and external health through energy healing, we can optimise our body, mind and environment for optimal flow, diminished resistance and complete acceptance of who we are. This allows us to focus on what matters – what our life purpose is and how can we fulfil this now. Only then, will we be truly happy and healthy.

"The Meaning of life is to find your gift. The purpose of life is to give it away."

~Pablo Picasso

About the Author

Dr Margo Livingston, an integrated medical consultant, has combined a unique and unusual skill set to create her bespoke 5 Pillars of Health, carefully designed to combine both western, traditional healing modalities with ancient eastern practices to offer her clients a 'Total Health Makeover'.

As an Immunologist, Advanced Nurse Practitioner, NLP Master Practitioner, Psychotherapist, and weight management, Qi Gong, Feng Shui and Bioenergetics consultant, with over forty years of training and experience, she has created a comprehensive therapy approach which guides people back to complete mental, physical and spiritual health and wellbeing. Margo recognises the essential but, often unknown need to interconnect both balanced inner body energy with that of the environment.

Dr. Margo runs a successful health consultancy globally online as well as face to face in both Spain and the UK.

You can reach Dr. Margo via her websites www.totalhealthmakeover.net or www.DrMargoLivingston.com or facebook page www.facebook.com/DrMargototalhealthmakeover or on LinkedIn www.linkedin.com/in/dr-margo-livingston-b0566ab5/

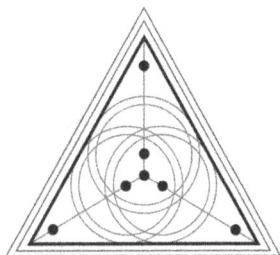

Part 2
Breaking the Cycle of Chronic Stress

Have you ever found yourself thinking that you would be so much more energized, so much more focussed, so much more YOU, if only you could detox from the stress in your life? If so, then that was your inner knowing talking, and it was absolutely right!

So much of our innate magic is just on the other side of fear, stress and anxiety. When we are tightly wound and doing a daily battle with our pain and everyday stressors, that's where most of our energy goes. The best version of our self, gifts and all, doesn't get to see the light of day.

But once we've healed from and moved past the peak of our trauma and stress, we find that our best self emerges. The talents we were born with, the purpose we came to Earth to pursue, our skills and our knowing all begin to bubble up to the surface.

The simple truth is that we can't fully actualize and live our best life while we are fighting a daily battle with toxic stress. Yet so much of modern society is fueled by stress — it's a tough problem to crack.

"The story of the human race is the story of men and women selling themselves short."

~ Abraham Maslow

Your inner knowing might already sense this, but let me tell you here that toxic stress is a viscous cycle. Becoming very stressed affects our mental and physical health, and alters how we respond to our world. Over time this turns into chronic pain and sickness, and a weakened level of resilience. This makes us more stressed, and so the cycle continues.

We don't break out of this cycle by staying where we are, accepting the toxic environment we are in, or by numbing the stress with short-term solutions. We break out by becoming conscious of the real problem, seeing further than those short-term solutions, and by being brave enough to make changes.

If you find yourself in a bad place right now, then I'm sure you already know that the answers do not lie in alcohol, pain killers, or any other addictive numbing behavior. And I hope you also know it is not a matter of 'toughening up' or 'soldiering on'.

Society rewards stoicism, but at a certain point this becomes unhealthy.

The Japanese culture for overwork and burnout is so ingrained in their society that they even have a common term for death by overwork — Karoshi.

I hope this shocks you to look at what you've unconsciously accepted as tolerable, because as a society we need to stop and ask ourselves what we have become. When did we start valuing working hard over our own lives? When did we take on the belief that we are not enough just as we are?

But there is more to this problem of toxic stress than the world of work. As humans we are susceptible to the effects of trauma lasting years after the event, in both our minds and our bodies. We hold stress in our brains, the tissues of the body, as well as our memories. Left unprocessed, this typically results in poor health. We may have anxiety, depression, inflammation, idiopathic pain, or all of the above and more. This is why self awareness and the willingness to work through our emotional pain is so important. Left unprocessed, we are simply simmering away in a toxic soup.

"Neuroscience research shows that the only way we can change the way we feel is by becoming aware of our inner experience and learning to befriend what is going inside ourselves."

~ Bessel A. van der Kolk, The Body Keeps the Score: Brain, Mind, and Body in the Healing of Trauma

As a physician focused on trauma healing, I want to bring awareness of this to as many people as I can possibly reach. We need to start being more gentle with ourselves, and respecting our need to grieve, process, and heal in our own time. But most of all, we need to stop avoiding what's going on inside ourselves, and start working through it, little by little in a manageable way.

In this section of the book you will hear from two authors who learned to process their stress and trauma, and who moved on in life to really embrace their gifts and live as their best selves.

In the first story you will meet Siv from Norway, who tells us how she healed herself from the physical damage stress had done to her body, enough for her to climb Mount Everest — twice. Siv had a stressful career that, being a good citizen and listening to society, she found hard to let go of. I'm thankful that she did finally give herself permission to choose another path in life, and is now happier and healthier for it. Like Siv, you may come to realize that it is often allowing yourself to finally put an end to a bad situation that takes the most inner work.

In the second story of this section you will meet Charlotte, who I've come to know very well over the years and am blessed to call a friend. Charlotte is an animal healer who has an amazing gift. But the catch is that this gift came from a near death experience, and the trauma of the accident that set her on this path almost prevented her from using her gift at all. Healing her original trauma and learning about how her body's stress response was affecting her was critical for Charlotte. Today she is following her life's purpose and using her gifts to heal animals, and this is such an inspiring outcome.

We all have gifts, but not all of us recognize this or notice what is special about us. I truly believe that when we are healed and our nervous system is calm again, this makes it easier for us to listen to our intuition and feel our way forward.

You may have picked up this book to learn about healing yourself simply in order to feel better. But I think you might also gain some insight into your own gifts as you progress along your healing journey. There is gold at the end of the rainbow.

Healing to Climb Mt. Everest

by Siv Harstad

It was Friday afternoon towards the end of June. The office was buzzing; people were happy for the great weather and that the weekend was starting. It had been a very busy day (week, month, year) and I had finally been able to sit down. As usual, I'd had a lot of ad-hoc activities, so all my planned tasks were on hold for later. I had a few minutes to check my email for any urgent messages before my next meeting.

Then Jacob, a colleague from a different department, came into my office. I had the role of Head of HR, so I expected he had something he wanted my help with. He sat down, looked at me and asked, "How are you doing?"

I smiled and answered, "I'm good."

He kept looking at me and said, "Yes, I know. But how are you really doing?" After a small pause, he continued, "I don't like that people are sick and don't come to work, but you need to talk to your doctor. I don't want to see you in the office on Monday."

I could feel the emotions coming up on the inside and I felt like crying. Deep down, I knew things were not good and had not been for a long time. I had done everything I could to keep going; ignoring all the signals from my body and making sure I was delivering all that was expected — and more. I was used to working a lot; however, what had been going on for the past few years was on a different level. I kept telling myself that it was not too long until my vacation and I soon would get the extra employee I had been promised for the past six months.

I had been so alone with all of this for so long. Jacob saw beyond the reassuring smile I put on. Tears were welling up in my eyes and started to roll down my cheeks. My voice cracked as I tried to joke it off and keep up my brave, "I'm all good" face. My emotions were shining through it all. I did not dare to fully feel how I was really doing. It was too scary. Because it was not good. I had this painful feeling in my chest and I did not want to, or dare to, fully feel it.

Jacob looked at me and told me, "This is serious. You have to take care of yourself. What is going on here is not good. Talk to your doctor and get some days off." He repeated that he did not want to see me in the office on Monday.

At the time, I did not fully understand what he said, or how bad things were, because I had been pretending I was all good. At that very moment, I did not think I needed to stay at home on Monday.

On Saturday, I visited my cousin who I had not seen for a long time. She's a positive, lighthearted person who is so great to be with. I had not been there very long before she asked me, "How are you doing?" Before I managed to say much, she continued, "and don't lie – I can see it in your eyes that there is something wrong."

I told her about the situation at work. Part of the environment was toxic and how it affected me, not sleeping and often not having time to eat lunch during the day. I had not realized how bad it had affected my body, because I had been reassuring myself I was all good and that it would soon be better. She told me: "You have to do something about this. Talk to your doctor and get a few weeks off."

Monday morning arrived and I was ready for work; dressed up and on my way to the bus. I had nearly arrived at the bus stop when I started to think, "Maybe they were right, maybe I should not go to work." I decided to go back home. Nearly back home I thought, "What are you thinking of? Of course, you are going to work." And down the hill I went again. Almost back to the bus stop, I turned around thinking I should not go to work. It all continued — up and down the hill five times. That's when it hit me — what I was doing was clearly not good. I decided to call my doctor.

A doctor in shock

The next day I was sitting in my doctor's office. I've had the same doctor for years, but had hardly been there. I told her what I was experiencing and she did some tests. When she saw how high my blood pressure was, she was shocked. She immediately forbade me from doing any physical training, except for slow walks. She explained that it would be dangerous for me to raise my pulse too high.

She gave me two weeks of sick leave. That would give me two weeks off of work, then straight into a two-week vacation. I felt like it was more than enough time and that I soon would be back at work.

Hidden illnesses and symptoms

During the following weeks, I had to adjust to a slow-motion lifestyle and found out it was not only the high blood pressure and not sleeping at night that were issues. I tried to read a book, thinking it would be a nice relaxing activity. It was impossible to read; I could not concentrate even if I tried. I had problems with my short-term memory and kept forgetting things. In addition there were health issues that had come up over the last six months that I had ignored: headaches, muscle pain, weight gain and a bad temper. I was behaving out of character and had pains I never experienced before.

I did my best to slow down; went for long walks since I could not train, caught up on sleep and prepared for the vacation. The two weeks went by fast. The vacation was an amazing trip with friends to East Africa. It was fantastic; however, the final week I did not sleep again. One of my friends noticed I did not look good, so while we were sitting at this beautiful location, by the pool, overlooking Lake Victoria, she asked what was wrong. I told her I was lying awake at night thinking about having to go back to work and that I was dreading it.

She said, "Siv, you don't have to get back to work" I looked at her in surprise. The idea had not even crossed my mind. "Are you sure?" I asked. She was sure and thought I should call my doctor when I got back. "If you are not sleeping then you are not ready to go back". The idea that this was even possible gave me some relief. I still did not sleep much; but it helped knowing that I might not need to return to work yet.

Acknowledging my toxic work environment

I had not told anyone how toxic part of the work environment was. Looking back, that was the worst part. It was very difficult because the company was great. I loved my role and like having lots to do. It was that other part that made it unbearable in the long run. I had briefly told two people about some of it and they both told me to leave. I dismissed it, told myself it was because of a specific difficult situation and that I could handle it. Truth to be told, none of us can stay in a toxic environment for long without being affected.

The journey back to health again

Back from vacation, I did my best to adjust to my new situation. My main focus was to become healthy and to get back to work. I went for daily walks and did all I could to improve my health. About one month after the vacation, I had a follow-up with my doctor and she sent me for some extra tests, to be 100% sure we were talking about stress and not a brain tumor or anything else.

One of the tests I took was a cognitive brain test. My brain was in general normal; however, they could see long-term effects of stress.

How crazy is that — stress was physically affecting my brain!? Stress apparently is one of the worst things we can do to our body. I had to admit that my burnout was severe.

Leaving what made me sick

As part of the sick leave follow-up, I met with the company I worked for and found out there was absolutely no interest in changing things at their end. It did not make sense for me to get healthy and go back to exactly what had made me sick.

I decided to leave the company. Signing an agreement to leave the company while on sick leave was a bad financial decision. From a mental perspective, it was one of the best decisions I have ever made. Such an unbelievable relief knowing I did not have to go back.

Climbing mountains

Climbing mountains is my big passion and before I got sick I had planned to climb a mountain called Ama Dablam in Nepal. I had been willing to leave my job to be able to go. Now, I had left the company, but had health issues. I discussed the expedition with my doctor. As long as my blood pressure was normal, I could go. In fact, she thought that it might even be beneficial for me to be in nature and have a totally different focus.

I was so grateful. A climb like this is a journey of a lifetime, on so many levels: nature, culture, people, friends, challenges, elements and being in the moment. I focused on taking things slowly and listening to my body — which is perfect in high altitude. It was tougher than previous high altitude climbs, but I summited — despite my fear of heights. What a victory it was standing on the summit of this exposed mountain!

Back at Base Camp, I was invited to come back and climb Mt. Everest. At first I said: "No thank you", like I had done three years earlier. I thought I did not want to climb Everest. My friend said: "Siv, if you want to, you can do it." I agreed to think about it and four months later, I decided "Yes!" Little did I know that Everest would be my main focus and reason to becoming healthy.

My big goal was now to climb Mt. Everest; a much fiercer goal than getting a new job. It would demand that I was healthy on all levels: mind, body and spirit.

Healing the effects of stress

My blood pressure was the easiest thing to cure. When I left the company, it went back to its normal healthy range and has stayed there ever since.

After six months, my short-term memory was improving and as I healed, my ability to focus and read slowly came back. Eight years later, I still read slower than before and have a shorter concentration span for certain things.

My energy remained very low; worse than in the beginning. Most likely because as my body finally relaxed and when it did I could feel its state, I could feel how exhausted I was. That's when I started to sleep a lot, my body was trying to catch up for lost hours. I remember that I three days in a row had slept 12 hours and all three days I needed the alarm clock to wake up. If not, I would have slept longer.

Sleeping

In fact, my biggest problem was sleeping and it took the longest to heal. I started using a sleep mask to get total darkness. To relax my mind, when I lay awake for hours, I found that meditation is what works best for me. Today, eight years later, I am still sensitive to light and I can sometimes feel my body needs a bit extra, so I allow myself 12 hours each night to get into balance.

Mindset

I literally met myself when I got sick. I had never been sick before and had thought to myself "How hard can it be to recover?" I found out. Not easy!

On many levels, a burnout is tougher than you think. I looked fine on the outside, but my body did not have any energy and my brain was not working like I was used to. It was hard to handle, not only my own expectations, but also other people who did not even remotely understand how I was doing.

I had to learn to rest during the day. For me to lie down on the sofa midday was a mental challenge, more than anything. I found a coach to help me adapt to my new situation.

Food and drink

The stress leading up to the burnout led to a lot of shortcuts and easy solutions with food. All in all, I gained about eight kilograms, despite working out. My body was in a constant fight and flight mode and wanted to keep all the calories. When I got sick, I became more interested in eating healthy and did everything I could to improve my health.

A few years earlier, I scanned myself on a biophoton scanner and started taking high-quality nutrients. When I got sick, my scanner score dropped significantly and got stuck for nine months. Nothing I did seemed to change it, until I did a 40-day juice fast with vegetables only. I felt amazing and finally my scanner score started to improve.

Training

When I started physical training, I had to think completely differently from before. I started very slowly, and gradually increased the amount and intensity. At times, it was very hard, because I wanted to improve fast. It was a constant pushing and holding myself back.

Another thing that was new and I had never done before was that I had to go home and rest, or even sleep, after my workouts. If I did not relax afterwards, I felt like I was hungover from a party the day after.

Everest ready

For a long period, the only things I focused on were eating healthy, nutrients, sleeping, training, acupuncture treatments and personal development activities. Everest was my long-term goal that I had my mind on and was working towards, on all levels.

In the Spring of 2015, two-and-a-half years after I got burned out, I was on my way to climb Mt. Everest. I knew I was ready — no more than that, I knew I could make it. I had climbed the sixth highest mountains before so I know what it takes.

Three weeks into the expedition, we experienced and survived, Nepal's 2015 major earthquake (7,9 magnitude). That day so much was lost in seconds. I am grateful I survived and nobody on my team was hurt.

The persistence and ability to push myself - to go the extra mile - was what made me push myself to the level I did. It was also what kept me going towards climbing Everest after the first attempt. I managed to finance the expedition again, train even harder and I went back in 2016. That time, I summited. On many levels, it was the ultimate test of fully recovering from stress and burnout. On a personal level, it was an amazing victory; especially managing to climb safely down when I became blind on the summit. (For more on that story, visit my website!)

My future looks bright

I am extremely grateful for experiencing the burnout and surviving the earthquake on Everest. They taught me the importance of balance in life and to listen to my body. These experiences have made me the person I am today — a better version of the one I used to be.

I am now planning some amazing expeditions to the poles and the world's most remote locations. I hold motivational talks and take people on fun and challenging adventures around the world. Perhaps someday I will help you achieve your 'Everst', too.

About the Author

Siv Harstad is an entrepreneur best known as an Adventurer and TEDx speaker. Siv is the first Norwegian woman to climb Mt. Everest from the Nepal side and one of the few hundred people on the planet to have climbed all of the 7 Summits (the highest mountain peak on all continents).

Siv loves reaching tough goals and helping others do the same. She is both an expedition leader, organizing eye opening trips for people around the world, and a motivational speaker using her background and skills to help businesses to develop and motivate teams to reach their "Everest".

Siv holds a Masters of Science in Business Administration (Siviløkonom) and has a corporate background as a Leader, Head of HR and a Consultant, with experience from Management Teams, large change and IT projects in both Norwegian and international companies. She is a certified NLP Coach and a Wilderness First Responder.

Connect with Siv directly siv@aimlofty.com or online
https://www.aimlofty.com/
https://www.instagram.com/sivharstad
https://www.facebook.com/AimLofty/

How Healing the Animals Healed Me

by Charlotte Banff

I never really gave much thought to the significance of the accident. After all, it had happened when I was very young, so I cannot remember my life as 'Before and After'. It has always been 'After'.

It took me 30+ years to figure out that there was something here for me to investigate, why diving into investigating this was actually significant for my wellbeing and recovery, and how it fit my purpose in this life.

So I started investigating! What had ACTUALLY happened, when I had been involved in a traffic accident, nearly died and left my body at age two-and-a-half?

In recent years, many more people have openly talked about their NDE's (Near Death Experiences) and OOB's (Out Of Body Experiences) and it's not a taboo topic any longer – hence, there's now much more material and information on the subject for me to investigate.

When I have read about people who had an NDE/OOB, it is very often with an emphasis on the difference for them between the life they'd had before the incident and then how that life changed after the incident. Many people can explain how the things they experienced changed their perspective on life. Many speak of having met angelic beings or an energetic presence of some sort and have received information and insights during their NDE/OOB that have given them a more awakened perspective on many things in their lives. Many have changed their whole life around after their experience by using what they learned to reshape their life.

Because I was so young that I barely remember anything from before the accident, this is not what I experienced. However, I still recognise that when an event like this happens, it must have some kind of impact. You cannot nearly die, leave your body behind and come back unchanged. It doesn't work like that! As this happened at such an early age, I do not have a comparison to bring into this equation of anything before the time of the event.

My motivation behind this long quest has been to understand the significance of this experience for me. I wanted to understand how my energetic body and my nervous system are constructed to enable myself to deal with the accident's effects.

So, *I* set up a list of questions for my investigation!

What actually happened to me?

What influence did it have?

What can I do with this knowledge?

Diving into the answers to these questions has been a journey of several decades, with answers and insights surfacing gradually, like peeling off the layers of an onion. The answers certainly did not just show themselves, simply because I decided to do some digging and investigate this further. These answers had to be lived out, they had to be experienced, in order to surface to my awareness.

I have experienced many healing crises since the accident, and there have been some 'dark nights of the soul' along the way, involving deep inner trauma work, to release the accident's impact on the physical, mental and emotional levels. It takes the time it takes because no trauma-release can be forced. It has to be met with patience, understanding and love.

I am fortunate because I certainly did not walk this path alone. I have definitely had some valuable assistance along the way – I have received wonderful support from many people and especially from a most beloved group of beings, who have turned out to be my friends, guides, helpers and mentors: The Animals!

Every time a healing crisis occurred and I had to relive the consequences of the accident, there they were, right by my side to guide me, help me and heal me; the animals, with their wisdom and insightfulness. They willingly and selflessly shared their love and *support* with me.

The story of a broken soul

'She did not know that she was allowed to connect to the Divine. They had taken that away from her! She knew that the Divine was where she should get her healing. Her body felt like a shell without life. She was robotically and mechanically eating and sleeping when she had to. Her body was running on instinct.

She was from Nature's hand and was a very connected animal, this stunningly beautiful, large, clever elephant.

As a species, she incarnated into this world to be with people and to spiritually uplift, educate and aid them in their transformation. But they never gave her the chance! They destroyed her. Broke her spirit. Took away her Divine Connection by the way they treated her and used her to their own benefit. Because this is often what people do to animals.

But she was saved and brought to an animal shelter. Because that is also what can happen to animals when they meet heartconnected people — and that's where we met her, connected our hearts *to* hers and helped her heal!

She had been at the rescue centre in Thailand for three months. Just eating, sleeping, and acting as if on auto-pilot. The keepers were worried about her. 'She has *sad* memories', *they* explained.

She accepted the Healing I offered. She started moving around in her pen. Her keeper noticed her change right in front of our eyes. Her keeper was crying from relief. We were all crying. She looked right at us and moved towards the gate to her pen, we could connect to her, she reached for us...

She was healed in her trust, that she was yet again re-connected to her Soul, as she was before she was broken. Integrated on spiritual, mental and physical levels, she was healed from there on, she could move on towards living an integrated life, for the rest of her time on this earth.'

What I do know for sure, is that what I experienced as a child, has primed my nervous system in such a way that I am able to use my nervous system and my energy body to reach into and read the subtle energies around me very clearly. I can channel and direct Source energy and healing to where I see it is needed, in both humans and in animals. And that's what I did for that elephant in Thailand.

My investigations into NDE/OOB experiences shows, that often people come back into their bodies with some heightened sensory abilities. For me, it is as if the 'filter' between the visible world and the invisible world around the animals is seamless. Like there is full coverage on the spirit-wifi for the animals!

My 'radar' for picking up energy frequencies is detailed. I can pick up from the animals what they are expressing non-verbally. This communication comes through to me in pictures, sensations and emotions. It comes as an internal dialogue with the non-physical world behind the animals.

I pick up messages, stories and subtle energies, broadcasted from their energy bodies and from the spirit world around the animals. I sense into the unseen energy layers of the Animal Kingdom and the expressions broadcasted from them.

What I needed to learn was how to navigate in this jumble of impressions within me; I needed to learn how to discern when I was being 'only me' or when something was present in my energy field that I was picking up from outside of me. It was not something that I could turn on and off, but it was just there in me as a shared part of my awareness.

'Just turn it off' was the reply in clinics I attended when I asked to learn how to master this 'gift'. That technique never worked because I cannot really turn off ME! So onwards I went with my investigation. I needed to find some kind of answer as to WHY I can do this, WHAT to make of it and HOW to put it to good use — as it certainly did not go away just by being told to 'go away"!

Oh, how I have struggled with this! All I wanted was to be 'normal' (what is that, anyway?) But that was what I wanted! Not to be so extremely sensitive, extra super intuitive and able to read e.v.e.r.y.t.h.i.n.g around me.

Even further, I just wanted to live in an 'earth suit' (a body), that worked! A body that would function properly and not have all sorts of extreme reaction patterns of pains and difficulties that made life *physically* and mentally challenging for me. I just wanted to have my body respond to life, like a 'normal body'.

Bouncing Back

'She was one of my first animal clients. I met her many, many years ago. A beautiful Soul. Zoe was a dog rescued off the streets in a country in southern Europe by a rescue organisation that was rescuing dogs and giving them a forever home with caring people

I met her because her new human friend wanted to give her *a* fresh *start* in life after everything that she had been through before her rescue.

She showed me what had happened to her. It was horrific to experience together with her how her life had been on the streets and what humans had done to her. She also had the physical scars to show for it. Her ears had fragments of gunshots and you could see burn-marks on her body. To me, it was inconceivable how she could feel any trust in humans.

However, as she lay there on her soft cushion, belly full, a loving human friend to share her life with and care for her, I learned a valuable lesson: You CAN heal from trauma and find some version of a loving and fulfilling life. When the right circumstances show up, healing IS POSSIBLE! Finding purpose out of a traumatised life IS POSSIBLE!

She walked The Rainbow Bridge a few years ago. I cried when I heard about her passing, but she got to become old and she was loved and had her human friend beside her until the very end. How blessed her life ended up being, despite how she'd started out. What if her life hadn't started out that way? She would never have met her human friend, *whom* she *gave* so much love and affection and shared so many special moments with. She influenced the life of her human friend immensely, just by her mere presence. And she taught me a most treasured lesson, that I now bring forth both in my own life and in the Healing Work I do for traumatised animals and rescue animals. Thank you Zoe, from my heart!'

To move forward, I needed to understand WHY my system was reacting and functioning the way it was and figure out how to make a life out of the hand I had been dealt.

Living in a traumatised body, with my nervous system constantly on high alert and an energy system constantly on a full wifi connection to everything broadcasting on 'Radio Spirit', has certainly been challenging for me in many ways. I have experienced multiple stress-reactions like break-downs as a result of the trauma. Stress responses in my body led to symptoms from autoimmune diseases, anxiety, nerve diseases, asthma, allergies, the list goes on. I also have a hearing disability that was caused by the trauma of the accident. As a child, I suffered from massive headaches and sudden strikes of pain in my head, because my head had taken such a blow in the accident.

The trauma of leaving my body behind had created a state of permanent fight-flight-freeze responses in my body. My system was holding on 'tooth and nail' to life. Our human bodies are designed to survive. To be able to do so, various functions in the body are prioritised towards keeping us alive. That often leads to other systems not functioning properly, as survival has top priority. Clever on some levels but highly inconvenient and frustrating on others!

Finding Flow

'I was in the rescue centre again, doing CranioSacral Therapy on the rescue animals. I have found during my own healing journey that this form of therapy is so soothing to the nervous system and it re-balances the body systems, creating a space of calmness, flow and healing. The animals love these treatments!

It was one of those days where I was not feeling my best but I needed to give him his treatment because he was certainly feeling worse than I was. I 'picked myself up' and did my preparations for the treatment, diligently taking the time I needed to *ready* myself so that I could give him the best possible treatment, despite the fact that I myself felt a bit 'off'.

I sat in his enclosure as I have done many times before over *the* last 10 years. We are friends now, me and him.

He climbed onto my lap and sort of just attached his body to my hands. He knows the drill. He knows the treatment I give him and he knows where on his body he needs the treatment the most. So I give him that. This is what I do! I can help him with this. I can hold a Space of Healing for him and soothe his path in life. I guess we hold each other, because my day is always 110% better when I have spent my day with Boris, the Red Vari Lemur.'

I have learned something very valuable along the way: There is no 'normal'! (So I have stopped chasing that, it appears to be a lost cause anyway!) There is whatever version of each of us, as represented by our very existence. This is unique and perfect, just as it is!

Because we all carry a gift from the Divine within us, we are all a unique fragment of the Source. This is how we can be unique individuals yet all have the same Source. When all the fragments are added together, the total energy sum of all humans is the Whole. We sum up to 1 = the One.

What we do to one another, we do to ourselves!

I have learned that despite whatever I may lack on the physical level, I can make up for in other ways. Because also persistence (which sometimes converts into stubbornness), resilience and perseverance lives in me…at least on the good days. And there are still 'not-so-good' days. But that is ok. I deal with those much better now. I deal with them from a place of being more connected and in more Faith. This, I believe, comes from having to hang on to life by the end of my fingernails and to work through a heavy layer of trauma. The effect is that I convert the experiences from early in life into something somewhat positive moving forward.

I believe that we are here on Earth, with all our uniqueness to be of service to that which makes us uniquely US and share that with one another. I am here to share exactly that, which makes me uniquely ME, quirks and all!

Everything I have experienced has served the purpose of making me ME, one way or another. Including that which I certainly would have liked to have been without. I would not have been ME without all of the experiences, again, quirks and all!

I am doing my best to put it all to good use by helping the animals of this world. Rescue animals are so desperately in need of help and healing from the way they have been treated in a human-dominated world. I see it as my mission to help them with what I can bring to the table, sharing ME, my experience and what that have taught me.

This is where I can use the results of my investigations. This is where it all comes together and makes sense, in some way. It gives me an immense sense of purpose! Because I KNOW IN MY BONES how it feels to live in a traumatised body. I KNOW how to soothe the trauma and hold the space for healing of a traumatised animal. Because I have walked this path myself and I have the ability to pass on this healing experience to the animals I work with. This is precious to me.

The Universe can be quirky, in a good way! I get to be best friends with some of the most endangered species on the planet. These animals trust in me, when I offer to share their stories and give them a voice. Sharing The Spiritual Voice of The Animals — that is my Mission!

Who knew, when I left school, that this would be my path – My plans back then were to be a professor in Latin and Greek – well, I guess The Universe had other plans for me...

About the Author

I'm here for the animals!

Charlotte Banff is a Lightworker for The Animals. She is CAO - Chief Animal Officer at Animalhealer Academy.

She lives with her husband (a lot of dogs, cats, chicken and horses … 😊) on their farm in Denmark. She loves connecting to Nature, growing vegetables and playing Gongs and Handpans — while also running an IT consultancy company.

Charlotte's mission is to broaden the awareness about the importance of the interconnectedness between humans and animals. How through healing, communication and consciousness work with animals, we can find a way to more compassion between humans and animals in the world we share together.

Charlotte is an ambassador for two of the largest rescue centers for animals in Denmark. She has founded the Animalhealer Academy and the hereto connected Animalhealer Academy Rescue Program, supporting the cause of Rescue Animals and their need for a respectable and decent life.

Connect with Charlotte:
www.AnimalhealerAcademy.com
http://www.facebook.com/AnimalhealerAcademy
https://www.instagram.com/animalhealeracademy/

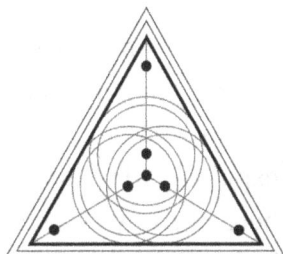

Part 3
Processing Grief and Trauma

In the worlds of integrative medicine and holistic therapies, we have long since understood that when we experience trauma, the body keeps a memory of it. If we have not processed a traumatic event, by coming to terms with it, finding meaning in the suffering or forgiving others and ourselves, if we have not found acceptance for what has passed, it is possible that the stored energy from the trauma will erupt in some way in the future.

Our pain has to show up somewhere, it has to be acknowledged and healed. If we don't allow that to happen in our minds, then the mental turmoil becomes a physical issue. This is often seen with survivors of abuse and other adverse experiences in childhood. In addition, growing up in a household where there was mental illness, alcoholism, emotional or physical abuse, abandonment, or having a parent who committed suicide or went to prison is associated with an increased risk of illness and behavior problems later in life. It is not surprising that there is a staggeringly high comorbidity between childhood trauma and a whole host of conditions and diseases including asthma, allergies, cancer, depression, fibromyalgia, chronic fatigue and other idiopathic conditions. (See the Reference section at the end of this book for our reference list, and take our Adverse Childhood Experiences quiz).

The body is a mirror of the subconscious mind. The traumatic experiences of life leave imprints in the mind, body and brain which later erupt in illness and disease. If we have help to process the traumas and dramas of life, the subconscious mind can retain the memory without a blemish on our future. We need a compassionate caregiver or person of authority to help us see that the abuse or attack we suffered was not our fault. We need to know that we are still good, worthy of love, and even when we were the ones to do wrong, we need to know that we can be forgiven.

But often, our parents and caretakers are not experienced in helping us make sense of the terrible circumstances of childhood. From being bullied at school, teased for our appearance, laughed at due to our speech or learning challenges all the way to the physical, emotional or sexual abuse we may have endured in childhood, the impact can last a lifetime without the therapeutic experience of being held with compassion, and listened to, heard and believed with openness. This is because being stressed or traumatized at a time when our brain was not fully formed, we did not have the capacity to comprehend the experience. So our tiny developing mind finds way to cope and makes associations between the abuse and our sense of self, and often in the most unempowered ways.

The emotional brain gets wired and programmed to find ways to survive. So we may take on beliefs and behaviors to shrink and make ourselves small, to tolerate even more unkind treatment. We may try to escape through dissociation, or numbing our pain with food, sex, shopping, drugs, or alcohol.

Unprocessed trauma through the eyes of the medical world

As a medical doctor myself, and one that has worked in both the traditional American hospital setting, and then later with Eastern Medicine as an acupuncturist, I am deeply fascinated by how the different areas of medicine and healing approach trauma.

From my own perspective, I honor the holistic, integrative approach and believe strongly that our psychology cannot be left out of the picture. What we were exposed to as children will have had a deep and lasting impact on our central nervous system. This is not an assumption, but a working understanding of neurodevelopment. When we are small children, we are in the most impressionable phase of our lives. Most of our learning about what the world is, and what we are here on the planet for, is formed in the first seven years of life.

During our first three years, looking at what our developing brain is doing holds the explanation for this. Our neurons are connected by synapses. The forming of these connections, to put it in the simplest terms possible, is what we call learning. When we see something new for the first time, our brain forms a synaptic connection, as we learn about this new thing. Now not every synaptic connection is made to last, and if we never see that thing again we may forget. But if we do see it again, then we have repetition of neural circuits, meaning our brain repeats the firing of electrical signals along that same synaptic connection the first time we saw that thing. Repetition is the key to reinforcing the learning and making something stick.

In practical terms, what that means for you is what you repeatedly experienced in childhood becomes a hardwired truth in your brain. If your caregiver repeatedly put you down, then you learnt low self worth. If your father repeatedly hit your mother, then you learnt that father-figures are dangerous. You can see how negative beliefs and fears are formed.

But what if you experienced a childhood trauma that was a one-off? Well, there is a caveat to this rule about repetition, as there is another way for your brain to define what is important and worth remembering. A trauma, especially something loud and scary, causes something called a 'flashbulb memory'. This is a single memory of an incident that burns so bright in its intensity, that you cannot forget it.

It will become encoded in your brain as a memory. It might be inaccurate, often flashbulb details are blurred by panic, but it will be there. It may not be remembered in a coherent order or with any words that you can recall, but there will be underlying emotions and perhaps a fear or anxiety that your central nervous system holds onto the memory of regarding the circumstances at the time.

If you've ever 'overreacted' to a loud sound or a particular situation, it may be that you have a memory you can't quite put your finger on, but your nervous system is triggered. As the stories in this section will show you, this isn't something you can outrun, mentally nor geographically. But it is something you can heal and recover from, when you are brave enough to face it head on and start to integrate all parts of yourself for true, holistic healing.

In this section of the book you will read stories of three women who learned, through painful life experiences, that not processing their emotions at the time of trouble, led to painful ruptures in body, mind and relationships later in life. You will also come to see how, even in our adult years, we can face those painful experiences and emotions, to put them to rest so that our body can heal and our mind can be free.

The first author we hear from is a wonderful trauma practitioner named Simone. Today she teaches meditation and coaches others through their own healing, but at the time of her story, she was deeply immersed in her own pain from a family issue. Using a healing conversation technique from a school of thought called Nonviolent Communication gave Simone the space and permission to process decades of pent up frustration she felt between herself and her sister.

These situations are not uncommon. How 'normal' is it for us to hold back complaints that we have with a family member so as not to rock the boat? Holding back the odd thing here and there might seem fairly innocuous, but when this becomes a habit or a way of daily life, the stress and frustration grows into something of a beast.

Trapped frustration, pain, stress or anger can take root in the body. As we already know, what we don't acknowledge and process mentally doesn't just get locked away in a neat little box, never to bother us again. What we repress will over time change from thoughts and feelings to physical manifestations of pain and disease. As to how that might manifest is completely unique to the individual — it could be inflammation, idiopathic pain, chronic fatigue, migraines, or something even more damaging.

What many people find is that when they finally stop repressing, and after the initial wave of emotion bursts out, things start to resolve themselves in a natural way. Finally processing what was pent up lets the body return to its natural state, and harmony can be restored in the body, the mind and the soul.

The next author you will hear from in this section is Cynthia. Her story is intense, and you will have no trouble seeing where her PTSD and Generalized Anxiety Disorder (GAD) originated from. While Cynthia's work at the time required her to speak publicly and give presentations, her body was doing battle with the PTSD and GAD, making her nerve-inducing speaking work an even more challenging task. The result of this was her central nervous system being in constant turmoil. This is a classic cause of inflammation and neurologic overwhelm in the body.

Experiencing a long list of painful and debilitating symptoms, but being able to rationalize them with her PTSD diagnosis, Cynthia pushed through them and continued to be in these situations at work. Over time this did more physical damage, and I think a lot of people could relate to this. Perhaps you have also pushed yourself harder out of a sense of duty, despite knowing deep down that what you really needed was to be kind to yourself and take a break.

Unfortunately society tends to favor those people who 'push through' and 'soldier on'. We are not rewarded for self awareness and self care in the same way, and this is a huge part of our problem the world over.

The bottom line is this. There is only one of you, and you cannot be present, happy or productive when you are stretched in too many directions. If you find yourself unable to move forward and progress in life, then take a look at what might be pulling you backwards. Those unprocessed, repressed traumas are often to blame.

The third story in this section is by a brilliant healer names Karin. As an adult she could trace back to her childhood an overwhelming sense of not being good enough. Early experiences with her father left lingering challenges with communication that she believed were also mirrored in her son.

Karin's story reveals the holographic nature of body and mind. What is left unprocessed in the subconscious will be mirrored in the physical world like a hologram. Fortunately a series of extraordinary spiritual and energetic experiences revealed ways to heal herself and the rest of the world too!

The Healing Conversation

by Simone Anliker

*'When someone really hears you without passing judgment on you,
without taking responsibility for you, without trying to mold you, it feels
damn good ... When I have been listened to, when I have been heard, I am
able to re-perceive my world in a new way and to go on.'*

~ Carl Rogers

Pain from the past

"What pain are you still carrying within you from the past?

Who is that pain connected with?

I will listen to you compassionately — stepping energetically into the
role of the person who you feel pain about.

At the same time, I will listen to you with an open heart, no judgments,
no blaming, no advice — being present with you empathically.

All you have to do is to speak out what is alive in you right now and
what arises in you when thinking of that person.

Don't worry about how to say it. Whatever way it wants to come out
is ok.

So who am I?" my coach asked me.

"You are my sister", I replied.

She took a deep breath and then asked me, "What would you like for
me to hear, as your sister?"

These were the opening words from my NVC (Nonviolent
Communication) coach, guiding me in my healing session which would
change my life and bring healing to a deep emotional pain I thought I
would have to live with for the rest of my life. They marked the

74

beginning of a journey of transformation not only for me but also for my sister. Within only two hours, I would go through a deeper transformation than I could ever have imagined being possible.

NVC as a life changer

Two weeks before this I had attended my first NVC intro workshop. I'd learned about NVC a couple of months earlier and had been struck by how this way of expressing and listening with compassion and love could help people to connect. I had been fascinated and immediately touched by this uplifting, life serving and deeply fulfilling awareness practice. I wanted to learn more about it.

During the course of the three days, participants shared their touching stories. I was quite 'successful' in holding back and controlling my emotions. But there was one woman who seemed to have a similar story like me. On Sunday morning, our last day of the retreat, she shared about her painful disconnect from her beloved sister. That was too much for me. I could no longer hold back. I burst wide open and started to sob and sob and sob. The dams were finally breaking. At that moment, I realized that pain itself decides when it's time to show itself. My time had come.

What I had tried to push away for years was now brought to the surface. Strongly, relentlessly! Pushing things away and pushing things aside are attempts to not feel something. It is equally true that exactly the opposite is the case. Resisting is persisting. Whenever I'd heard a similar story or whenever I'd seen a similar situation on TV, the pain had been there. So here it was in all its intensity.

Time to heal

I was ready to do anything if only the suffering would stop. I did not have access to my sister at the time. An open, honest conversation with her seemed impossible to me. This Sunday morning, my coach suggested having a Healing Conversation.

Two weeks later the two of us met. In a 'role play' of a special kind, she slipped into the role of my sister. She did not pretend to be her but dove into her energy, similar to the approach in a family constellation session. But rather than roleplaying, she was role-being. In this unique Healing Conversation, the coach is the substitute of the person of concern. What was special was that she was energetically my sister but at the same time listened with an open heart with full presence, empathy and compassion — so she was actually in a double role being the coach and fully participating in the healing.

I was invited to talk to her in a direct way while imagining that I was talking to my sister. Everything on my mind and in my heart was welcome to be expressed completely in an unfiltered way. All my pain, my anger, my sorrow and despair, my hurt, my grief, my disappointment, my mourning, my regrets, all my questions of why and how all this had happened, all there were allowed to be expressed and at the same time, were heard and received by my sister (through the coach) with an open heart, without the slightest bit of judgment or blame, with presence, empathy and compassion. Once in a while, she reflected back feelings and needs, which assured me that I had truly been heard and understood.

Unconditional listening

Never in my life before had I been able to express myself so fully yet at the same time been received so completely. I remember that in the beginning, I had still held back. There were things I didn't want to say, things I had never told anyone before. Every now and then I became aware that I was actually talking to the coach. I held back certain things because of shame, fear of rejection, of hesitation of what the coach might think about me. However, again and again, she asked me, 'Is there more you would like me to hear?'

My resistance melted, my courage grew and I allowed myself to free myself from all the burden that weighed me down. Even as I write this, I feel tears of gratitude filling my eyes and my heart. What a gift it is to have someone listening to you and holding you with such care while you are revealing yourself with all your shadows and woundedness!

This part of the Healing Conversation lasted about an hour until everything had been said and all had been expressed that wanted to be expressed. I remember how liberating and freeing it had been and how light I had felt after being received without the slightest judgment.

After about an hour, there had been nothing left in me that had needed to be added, mourned, explained or asked. My sister (coach) had then asked me if I was ready to hear how she was feeling with all that she just heard.

Time to reconcile

Yes, I was ready now — finally ready to hear my sister.

It was amazing to me how easy it was to listen to her as the way she expressed and honored my feelings and needs opened the way for me to connect with her.

I was astonished by how the coach had picked up wordings and ways of expressing things exactly as my sister would have. It really felt like sitting in front of her. She was morning and regretting her actions after listening to how her behavior had affected my life and thus I was able to empathize with her. She expressed what was going on in her and why she had interacted with me the way she had. My heart was melting and I was willing and able to empathize with her. The magic of mutual connection and reconciliation took place. I suddenly was able to see both sides. Deep understanding and a feeling of love were rising in me. I felt such a relief. And things changed.

Change the way you look at things and the things you look at change.

~ Wayne Dyer

I hadn't known this quote at that time but it is definitely true for me now. With the help of this Healing Conversation, I was able to change the way I looked at my story and relationship which literally changed my relationship with my sister.

The pain is gone

Immediately after the Healing Conversation, I felt much more relaxed around her. I remember that my coach asked me to do some kind of work after our session — maybe writing or awareness practices but the fact is, I forgot about it completely. I felt such a relief and such a weight was taken from my soul that nothing was left in me that needed any attention around that pain anymore. The pain was gone! Being heard completely, and I really mean completely, left no trace, no word that wanted to be expressed or added to what had already been said.

During the month after that, I felt the enormous power and transformation of the work we had done. My relationship with my sister normalized. We very naturally grew closer again and it opened the door for a scary, totally honest, and raw conversation about two years later that led to the true friendship of soul sisters again. I could not even have dreamed of such a change.

Learning the magic

After my healing transformation, I decided to become an NVC trainer. I especially wanted to learn this healing practice. I was fascinated by the effectiveness and power of it. Even though it needs a high skill level of presence, compassion, detachment, letting go and letting in God, I am convinced that most of us have the ability to become healing coaches. I started to teach it.

One of my clients, a naturopath, used this practice as a way of communicating with her patient's organs. As a coach, she represented her client's organ and invited her patient to have a direct conversation with the organ. I liked her creativity and she was quite successful in helping people to reconnect with their bodies.

Having done a lot of Healing Conversations over the years, I find it interesting that normally I don't remember a lot of details. It is part of this unique healing technique that I am there as the coach, holding my client with care, and at the same time, I am stepping aside while I open energetically to the person I connect with. I am part of the process with a dual awareness.

The following are two of my clients' stories. Even though both of them were aware of my being the coach representing their beloved ones, what they remember from these conversations is a direct interaction with their beloved ones and the shift in energy, emotion and awareness.

Eva's story

'My son committed suicide in 2011 without leaving a letter. The only thing he left was a note saying, "I don't want to be re-animated."

We didn't understand why. We knew he'd been in physical pain since his car accident seven years ago but we thought he'd been doing all right.

When you and I met, I was in intense emotional pain and very worried if he was okay wherever he was. Our Healing Conversation was so helpful. Right at the beginning, you told me that there is so much love emanating from him. This in itself was deeply calming for me. Through you, he told me that he was okay and that he knew that I was able to forgive him. "Don't worry!" he said to me. As a mother that was very important for me to hear. I asked him if he wanted flowers and candles on his grave as we normally do in Russia. He told me that if that is important and soothing for me then I should do it. I realized that it wasn't important to him.

Between his accident and his passing, there had been seven years. In this time he had gone back to school, graduated from high school and started university. He told me in our Healing Conversation how important this had been for him and that he'd wanted to do this. You told me all this without knowing him. It was obvious to me that you were in connection with him. You did not know about all that.

I was so happy that he was still somewhere around and that I'd had a chance to communicate with him. I knew that wherever he was, he was fine.

After our Healing Conversation, I felt changed. I didn't have to cry so hard anymore. I was calm and I felt completely different. I am still so grateful. You really helped me a lot.

Even years later when I felt down, I could go back to this conversation and find peace in me again. If it hadn't been for this conversation, I wouldn't have had any chance to connect with him again.'

She then added, 'Can you see how calmly I am talking about all this now? I am also so fortunate that I know all about reincarnation. I believe that he is already back here in a physical body again. If I'd only had the knowledge of the Catholic church that would have been really hard. They told me that he is in hell, but I know better.'

Jolanda B's Story

'I was the child that no one wanted. I'd always felt that. My mother had never stood up for me. So I left home when I was 16 and did not come back to visit. I unconsciously blamed her.

In our Healing Conversation, I realised that she hadn't been able to behave differently. I felt it. I suddenly had some understanding of her as I was able to listen to her (through you) on how she was feeling. She explained to me how it had been for her. She had not been able to stand up for herself in her relationship with my father thus she had not been able to stand up for me. This had helped me to accept her thoroughly without accusation.

The Healing Conversation also changed her relationship to me. I could feel her deep joy and gratitude until she died. A peace has arisen in me. It even influenced my relationship with my own children.'

There is hope for you, too

"If you still carry pain about a person you lost connection with or you don't have access to, there is hope. You can free yourself from that pain and find peace. "

About the Author

Simone Anliker, LL.M., is a Certified Trainer for Nonviolent Communication, a certified NARM Trauma Practitioner, iEMDR coach, author of The Power of Dyad Meditation and co-author of several other books. Simone is owner of Compassion & Voice which is an international seminar and coaching company based in Switzerland.

Simone trains internationally as a transformational and meditation coach. Her interest is in spiritual NVC, psychology, healing and transformation.

In January 2017, she founded TheGlobal Dyad Meditation Project, a world-wide conscious online community that connects people, no matter where they are on the globe, through a unique, powerful meditation process, called the Global Dyad Meditation Process.

Get in touch:
Simone Anliker
Life Coach – Trauma Work
CH-6052 Hergiswil

Switzerland
info@compassion-voice.ch
www.compassion-voice.ch
www.globaldyadmeditation.org

Runaway Pain!

by Cynthia J. Harrison

Her body froze as she saw him coming in the hallway. She had nowhere to turn or hide. She took a deep breath and kept going. She can't recall words, but can still see his face. He was calm and seemed almost free from the demons that had tortured and engulfed his existence.

He was getting help, she trusted that was enough. Her superiors were alerted to his struggle, and concerns around how he would desperately grasp at her, or sit and watch with frightening intent, struggling to live with the choices he had made. He knew most would never forgive him and in his mind, she held the key!

Broken yet mechanically doing what she could to survive and care for her children, she soldiered on. Turning off emotions and feelings, she robotically did what was required of her. She was a shell of herself, having to swallow her emotions. There was no room for sustenance. Each time she ate she felt sick, like a monster in her belly was rising up, spitting fire in response.

Investigations were happening in the background. Her lips were sealed to protect others. She was told this was the only way to help the victims of his crime. Yet in the silence she wanted to scream, to roar like a lioness in his face and shake him to his core.

"Stay in centre" she would tell herself, "chant, stay with self", chanting Om mani padme hum as many times as it took – she had to play the role and it was slowly killing her.

He was her love, and she in a twisted way his, yet life had dealt a mortal blow to their connection. A shadow had crossed his path, and he saw no light in that darkness. Society would not allow him to be in her life. And she had to choose her own path.

She's here!

"I found her!"

A sergeant yelled from the pioneer's training room.

She looked up stunned.

The turmoil of many running and yelling "she's in here" electrified the space.

"Me?

Why?" she asked.

They looked relieved, like they could finally take a breath – now that they found her – alive.

She wondered about her family, screaming out loud "What? WHAT!" Later realising the men had thought she may be dead!

Let's go back a little

She held the role of Company Quarter Master in the Defence Force, overseeing the running of the stores with responsibilities for non infantry support roles. That afternoon she issued the weapons to the soldiers, they cross referenced the serial numbers and signed for their allocated rifle. She locked the armoury and got on with her tasks of inspecting and testing equipment serviceability.

The chainsaws and jack hammers were next on the list, and with Pioneer Platoons assistance they started up and ran the equipment. With this orchestra of industrial sounds coupled with the wearing of hearing protection, we were not aware of the disruptions happening just on the other side of the door.

He did it!

He had done it! He had released himself from his self made torment. Using the weapon she issued him, he had shot himself in the head. Planned down to the last theatrical piece, he had forgotten his helmet and had to go home to get it. It was a key part of the plan and couldn't be left out. The letter said it was to catch his brains so as not to make a mess. He wanted her to have the helmet for the mantlepiece to remember him. Morbidly romantic.

Thank goodness he left a note, a manuscript really, many pages long, and also a scribbled note for the first responders to see. He had thought of everything, except how to live.

All were questioned that night and she was shown the note. I'm not sure she could even read it. Shock of a near miss mixed with the loss, horror, and sadness that he was gone in such a way. It made her body tremble. The police protected her from seeing the body, and she was thankful for it. She was sure her mind's eye would have burnt the image into her vision for life.

They turned

The mood eventually changed from shock and disbelief, to anger and judgement. Many of his friends and family contacted her for support. She consoled them, while holding in her own feelings and the deeper truth of the "why" that he meticulously wrote out for her. His family were looking for answers and thought she could enlighten them. As they learnt more about their son the anger started, and the why's got more intrusive. It became uncomfortable to go to work. Her university studies began to suffer. Her body also reacted to the further turmoil. She developed Post Traumatic Stress and General Anxiety Disorder. The world hit her hard!

Run for recovery

It was decided! We would leave, pack up our entire lives and go to the other side of Australia to recover and start a new life. Run away really, any opportunity to escape the inescapable. Leaving her career, study and research opportunities, to merge into being just another looking for work in a new state where she knew no one.

The expression of grief was not fully possible due to the unresolved accusations of crimes he would not be held accountable for in life, yet he had admitted to in death. Blame started to turn towards her, and her own feelings of guilt and responsibility that she could have done more to help everyone grew. Yet the complexity of the investigations meant she had to keep her distance. Play her roles and just keep doing what she had to do to keep her household together. Work and study to stay distracted. Her body had other ideas.

Her ability to stand and speak in front of people was in combat with her nervous system. She would sweat so profusely it would trail down her whole body in a tickling motion. In constant survival mode she battled it by wearing clothes like jumpers to disguise and absorb it, winning tiny conflicts within, but not the war in full deployment on her nervous system's health. It became so uncomfortable being in her own skin that she became skilled in the ways of getting out of particular jobs and tasks that put her front and centre or in the light.

Anxiety kept her feeling small, out of control, and not fully in her truth or body. This added to the shame, guilt, and frequent thoughts of not being good enough that became symptoms of her ongoing terror. Prior to a work presentation she would feel nauseated and have diarrhea, perspire, and a dry cotton mouth through it, afterwards she would feel sick often ruminating over her performance. No one seemed to notice. With such expectations of herself, and coping tricks as a disguise, I guess her high functioning masked a lot of the symptoms.

As time went on

She would experience debilitating conditions such as memory loss and stammering. She would lose her words and train of thought. Migraines, sleep problems, fatigue, sweating, skin problems including an unexplained rash on her neck, acne, blurred vision, vertigo, nose bleeds, aches and pains, flash backs, tremours, hair loss, heart palpitations, and chest pain to name a few.

Ignoring and shutting herself off as a survival mechanism, she was to develop many discomforts, and her subconscious screamed to be heard through the physical body. The body was keeping tabs, reminding her daily of what she wished to be different, yet felt out of her control. Doctors were uncertain of what her body was manifesting and they all wanted to prescribe medications to numb her even further, but she refused. That felt like a further silencing of what they hadn't already heard or understood of her systems.

What she needed was a way to speak to and understand her nervous system. The practice of what she went on to teach via the healing arts. A way to be in her body, with her Self, which allowed the small voice within to be heard, and the nervous system to heal.

Toxic stress

Swallowing her deep suffering, her heartbreak, the confusion, and disbelief of how this beautiful soul could dive so deep into the realms of hell, never to return. No one could have saved him. She eventually understood that it was his own journey, as it was part of hers.

She would try to move and release the build up of toxic stress chemicals building within her by walking, running, or lifting weights. Until one day something felt very wrong. Her neck felt compromised and she was dizzy. The doctor said, "You can go home but you could be dead in 30 minutes. Your choice!" So she went to the hospital for tests.

She recalled her distress as the doctor attempted to do a lumber puncture (spinal tap), trying to be still as the sobs reverberated through her body. Feeling the morphine move through each part of her vein, cold as it moved up her arm and into the rest of her body. The gentle loss of control, so sensitive, even while trying to be numb to the world.

With neurological checks every hour, they kept her in for two days. Under surveillance, the impact of the muscle and soft tissue injury was not due to a stroke or an aneurysm as they thought. Instead it was just another load of unnecessary stress to stack upon her mind and body, not to mention her family.

On a daily basis it was if a new trial surfaced just to test her. Just to see how much she could withstand. She was really starting to break down physically. Mindfulness meditation helped but was not enough. Her suppressed rage and suffering could not be silenced. It had its own language and it burst out onto her face unexpectedly. The energy needed a voice, a way to be heard, not just calmed. Keeping it in was like someone saying to you when you're upset to "calm down dear!" Behaviour is a language and if we don't have or know the words our body will speak for us.

Dermatologists gave her medication that she was allergic to and this created large cyst like eruptions that scarred her face. Her lips blew up, filling with liquid. So now her external self was just as scared as her heart. Each day she saw her reflection, she was reminded of what she was trying to run from. Her mere presence was the reminder. How was she to love this vehicle that held the markings of all that she tried to forget?

On many occasions she would wake up crying out WHY! Why did she have to struggle and do her practice just to get up each day. Why was it such an effort just to get through a single day? Why, when she would have a disagreement did thoughts of that person harming themselves come in? Or driving home to her partner, why would flashes of finding him dead come to mind?

She was haunted by the past. It had taken much of her youth, her freedom, her looks, her joy, and her health. However, she would fight. And by doing her individual practice each day, she would come to understand how to not allow another's actions to define her any longer.

She can breathe!

To fully recover she left all she had built yet again and moved to Botswana, another opportunity to leave the world and reset herself (and her nervous system) outside of the stressful culture her profession entailed her to be part of.

Her roles over the years as a social scientist (social worker/ anthropologist) was direct work with oppressed and abused adults and children, witnessing and holding their pain for healing and empowerment. Creating space for hope, she loved being with people. As a sensitive individual she felt and absorbed her clients pain, and they would walk away lighter, thanking her. Though she felt a sense of satisfaction in helping others, she was left with a growing weight of suffering that accumulated inside her. She hadn't yet learned a healthy way to release and move past this unfair trade of emotions.

It was as if she fell into roles that perpetuated her experiencing of abuse, death, and disempowerment. She was trained in complex trauma both formally and via her own life experience, yet it seemed her life was to be at the col face, the razor's edge, all adding to the daily adrenaline and flood of cortisol. Understanding she needed a change, she chose to take an opportunity to do research in Botswana.

Learning how to use the earth to ground her body's electrical charge and keep the energy systems strong and in alignment made all the difference to how she could work in service to others and also herself.

She remembered feeling safer in Africa than at home in Australia. It was like the land, animals and people were healing her.

Already a spiritual woman who had practiced alternative health and wellness most of her adult life, she met a soul sister who became her dearest friend. They went on drives into unknown places in Southern Africa and shared wisdom with elders and people along the way. While sitting having tea, they were randomly invited to participate in a breath training that would add the structured pieces she needed to fully heal and gain her power back.

Time in her own body and breath to inspire. It became a place to learn to breathe fully in and fully out once again.

She was blessed

She can recall as she learnt to breathe, she would feel the subtle energy flow. By the end she felt the strings of energy lines streaming out from her fingers into the universe. As she asked what was happening she was told by the beloved teacher that she was blessed. That's it! That was all she needed to be reminded of. She was blessed.

On return home she continued her daily practice and she was now an expert at regulating the many arms of her nervous system. As she spoke to someone and her pulse raised to 108 just standing there, she would gently take control and breathe herself back to homeostasis. This is a way to say to the self "you're ok, there is no threat."

She dove into energy work in an even deeper way, now that she could feel and see it, studying with many spiritual teachers and energy masters, learning subtle energy functions, specifically those activated in a trauma response.

Her practice kept her nervous system steady to continue work with vulnerable people. She now had ways to hold space for their healing, keep boundaries and earth her charged energy in order to do and be more of who she is. Now rather than taking on their pain and suffering she would sit in the fire with them, showing the way through and out. Guiding as she held the story and its energy, she had been to the darkest shadows and could now support others in their journey home to Self.

Sharing her wisdom

Her symptoms were to dissipate over the first year. The practices built upon each other, allowing her to experience vibrant health with a deep understanding of both the physiological and energetic arms of the nervous system. She learned how to drive the body vehicle, but more importantly how to maintain and service it for optimum performance, like a high performance racing vehicle!

Allopathic medicine was and is a blessing, yet what healed her and her soul were holistic methods, the mastery of the breath with creativity, and energy medicine.

Stepping fully into her role as a medicine woman with many modalities, culminating her own wisdom and knowings into her current field of practice, she now speaks on stages and platforms to thousands of people. She does this with literally no stress response, and no anxiety. Her system knows it is safe and is no longer triggered by the past.

The tight rope she walked daily became the place of centre, seeing the polarity of life's ebb and flow from the neutral mind. She was able to love others from this space, but her greatest lesson was to deeply love her own Self. This achievement led to complete healing and helped her put to rest the ghosts of the past.

Forgiving all, including and most importantly herself.

Cynthia J Harrison

About the Author

Cynthia Harrison is the Founding Director of Rhombus Healing Arts in Perth, Australia. She is a Bio Field Science and Eden Energy Medicine Certified Practitioner, with degrees in Anthropology, Social Work, and Visual Arts.

Specialising in human behaviour she focuses on the evolution of the human, physically and energetically – offering a complete mind, body, spirit experience. The key to Cynthia's work is the overlaying of physiology with the energetic understanding of stress and complex trauma for conscious evolution. Knowing how the nervous system responds and behaves as a result is core to many illnesses, diseases, and discomforts.

An inventor and visionary artist, she creates interactive opportunities for wellness education and self empowered healing experiences. When not travelling to share the work, you can find Cynthia in her studio/clinic serving humanity to assist overall wellness for optimum vitality!

To support your nervous system health and wellness go to
www.rhombushealingarts.com

for tools and techniques. Or
www.facebook.com/Rhombushealingarts/

Instagram @CynthiaJaneHarrison

From a Hole in the Heart to Wholehearted Expression

by Karin Eke

I had always been hard on myself. Right from the beginning. It was as if I were punishing myself for coming into physical form and not being the perfect person that the world was waiting for to create peace on Earth! Growing up, I often felt frustrated that something was missing, without being able to express this or even understand it. As far back as I can remember, I was never enough and nothing I could ever do, say or be could satisfy my unconscious desire to be more. Not to mention satisfy my insatiable father, or at least that's what I felt at the time.

Having said that, I grew up in a relatively peaceful environment. All my material needs were met and most of my childhood was plain sailing. However, my inside world was at times a completely different scenario. My emotional needs were often left unattended, and allowing others to trample all over my feelings became my norm. To be honest, I didn't even know that my feelings were important and whenever I felt upset or unfairly treated, I would remain silent and push these feelings away. I had learned to make myself emotionally uncomfortable so that everybody else could feel emotionally comfortable.

To illustrate this, the memory of which I have absolutely no conscious recollection, my father would put his arms around me at a very early age and prevent me from moving while I was being fed so that I wouldn't make a mess. Had I already put myself into a straight jacket? I can only imagine that being restrained in my movements led to my feeling completely inadequate and out of alignment with my true self, that I had no right to express myself freely and that I had no other choice but to surrender to my parents' greater power. Whatever it was, very early on it no doubt shaped me into silence, frustration and a feeling of non-existence. This became a common theme throughout my life showing up in various different circumstances.

Communication was the title of one of my favourite songs as a pre-teen in the early 80s. Little did I know at the time that I was resonating at a deep level not only with the words but with the beat of the song as well. I was dancing to the ballet of Spandau Ballet and I was already in my own prison, my own self-created Spandau prison.

The communication issues first showed up during my teenage **years,** as far as I can recall, when communication broke down between my father and me. I didn't know how to communicate with him and certainly didn't have the tools to improve the situation. Neither did my parents. I felt trapped in an impossible situation.

The Pattern Repeats Itself

The plot was to thicken yet again many years down the line. In 2001, I was absolutely devastated to learn that my son, Thomas, had congenital heart disease. The old communication story was back in full force, as one of the diagnosed anomalies was inter-ventricular communication, meaning that he had a hole in between the ventricles of his heart. At the time, I just knew that my son was bringing forth a message for me, but I couldn't quite understand it. What's more, he was born just before 9/11. My son's arrival definitely shook up a lot in my life. Disbelief on hearing the diagnosis when I was 5 months pregnant, and disbelief again on hearing about the 9/11 incident. Oh yes, that feeling of disbelief was familiar to me and took me back to a heart-wrenching moment many years previous when my first boyfriend had wanted to put an end to our relationship. The feeling was showing up again, the emotion, the energy in motion that was still trapped within me.

Thomas, which funnily enough means twin, had open-heart surgery at birth and we were told at the time that he would probably not be able to survive without a second operation before he was 1. His heart had 3 major malformations: transposition of the great arteries, coarctation of the aorta and interventricular communication, but he had a choice, and he had obviously decided to thrive.

Magically and much to my relief, his heart adapted to the situation, just as my heart magically adapted to the situation of the heart-breaking and chaotic divorce I experienced a few years later. Our 'twin towers', which I saw as a metaphor representing the feminine and masculine figures, were destined to crumble, leaving a lot of debris.

A Huge Opening

In 2010, Thomas led me towards a deeper understanding of life. He was seeing a therapist as we couldn't understand some of his behaviour. I was absolutely amazed as these sessions had an immediate knock-on effect on me as I suddenly realised how interconnected we are. He was dealing with his emotions and my energy had been set in motion! I started having many beautiful, magical and mystical experiences beyond anything that I could possibly have imagined. It was like going through a portal to an infinite and parallel universe.

My first mystical experience was absolutely breathtaking. I was woken up early one morning and lifted out of bed by some immeasurable force that felt extremely loving and invigorating. We were expecting visitors that weekend and I had forgotten to set my alarm. How relieved I felt to have been woken up naturally at the perfect time in order to accomplish everything I needed to that day!

I felt as though I had a divine, invisible team working with me. The events of that particular day were all divinely orchestrated. It was as if my body knew precisely what to do next to create the most exquisite day for everyone, including myself. My to-do list became redundant as I was being guided all the time, my thinking mind had been overtaken and I simply glided from one activity to the next with ease and grace.

How surprised and excited I felt while preparing the dinner! It was as if somebody or some force had taken control of my hands and arms and the vegetables were being cut up for me and through me. There was absolutely no doubt that I was in an expanded state of consciousness and in universal flow. I felt light, expansive and ecstatic.

I existed in this expanded state and on top of the world for months. At times, I really couldn't believe what was happening as everything just became so easy. That summer I was intuitively guided to Louise Hay's work and came across her book You Can Heal Your Life. I felt so excited reading it that I couldn't put the book down. I had eczema at the time and I excitedly looked up the deeper meaning of this condition. When I read that the old thought patterns associated with this skin disorder were 'breathtaking antagonism' and 'mental eruptions', I was filled with astonishment. I was having unconscious mental eruptions and this was showing up as eruptions on my skin in the form of red, itchy patches! Wow, I thought. It was a pivotal moment for me as I realised the connection between our mind and body and the power of our thoughts. A few months later, I realised that I no longer had eczema and hadn't had any symptoms for a while. I had freed myself from this condition by freeing myself from my pent-up emotions.

Being in this flow state led me that same year to an out-of-body experience while visiting my parents on a family holiday. I directly experienced that I am so much more than a physical body, that I am not my body. I completely saw through the illusion of my reality. It was as if I were in different dimensions simultaneously, being the observer of my life on the one hand, and fully participating in it on the other. When I came back down to Earth with a thud a couple of days later, I felt like this infinite consciousness had trouble fitting back into my body. I knew that life would never be the same again.

Chaos and New Order Simultaneously

In 2013 and amidst a challenging divorce, a new door opened to energy healing and a whole new world of experiences started to unfold. It was as if I were back in Wonderland with yet more magical adventures. On running energy after my first Quantum-Touch workshop, the energy healing modality in which I later became certified, I was so astounded when my hands disappeared. This left me in complete awe as all I could see was energy and it was yet another confirmation of our infinite potential. The magic didn't stop there either. I healed an open and bleeding wound in a matter of minutes a few months later and even had a rejuvenation experience, where it was as if I were back in my 18 year-old body! I can only describe this as connecting deeply to my Higher Self when I allowed Source energy to run through me. As I write, I can feel energy rushing into my body as if to confirm the truth of this. I truly believe that this is how powerful we can all be when we are in touch with this greater part of ourselves.

Life was truly showing me how we create our own reality and I set out on a mission to explore consciousness, share how limitless we all are and how we have the power to heal ourselves from any dis-ease.

However, the obstacles didn't stop there. Another wake-up call was to rear its head in 2018. Never in a million years did I think I was going to receive the diagnosis of MS. There was no family history of chronic illness of which I was aware and I had spent most of my life in what I thought was a healthy body. My immediate reaction was to question the diagnosis. 'Oh no, how am I ever going to get myself out of this fine mess I've got myself into?' I jokingly thought to myself as my heart sank. Once again, this was a familiar feeling that was coming back with different circumstances, that feeling of not being able to escape from a situation, of feeling trapped, including past traumatic experiences of sexual abuse.

However, there had been signs of it for a while that I hadn't understood at the time. My mother was looking after a lady crippled by MS and unable to move without assistance. Deep down within me, I knew that this lady didn't have to be that way, that the illness could be reversed. It was nevertheless frustrating for me not to be able to articulate that in a way that could be heard. Frustrating because I was also emotionally involved in the circumstances, otherwise it wouldn't have triggered a reaction within me. Having the awareness that whatever I see projected onto the 'screen' of my life which reactivates an emotion within me is always reflecting something back to me enables me to expand, opening a door to transformation.

I am now excited to be able to share the good news that I have started to reverse the disease as the latest MRI scan results show that one of the lesions has completely disappeared. From my point of view, one of the keys to healing is associating our feelings and emotions triggered by current circumstances with similar feelings from the past, as everything is energy in motion, coming back in a different way in order to catch our attention ... to release the tension.

I believe that there are many different paths for looking at healing. My experiences have shown me that when I release emotions, I also release the associated physical symptoms and I naturally vibrate at a different frequency. This can be illustrated with the case of eczema as after just one healing session with me, my mother, who has had eczema for as long as I can remember and who is very sceptical about the work I do, healed completely from this condition. When we heal the root cause of any illness for ourselves, we can naturally help others achieve the same because we affect our environment and beyond with our own vibration.

As far as I can tell, chronic illness can only ever come from chronic stress of which we're often completely unaware. It can be uncomfortable dealing with it, which is why I pushed it away unconsciously. However, once we do deal with it, the breakthroughs are beyond our wildest imagination. I believe that our body is a holographic projection of our consciousness, sending us messages to help us evolve. We can directly influence this hologram with the power of our thoughts, intentions, feelings and emotions, thus enabling us to have complete control over its physical health. Our minds and hearts are truly powerful tools.

One of my visions is to see the end of pain and suffering for every living being on Earth and see everyone living in a permanent state of joy and bliss, simply because I've experienced this for myself. Being in tune with our intuition and following what brings us joy, however illogical that can seem, are also important keys to healing. I also truly believe that we live in one big cosmic joke and we can all be considered as clowns playing our role on the stage of life. We get to choose whether the play in which we perform is a comedy or a tragedy. I know which one I've chosen. For me, laughter is the best medicine. What about you?

About the Author

Karin is a lightworker, mystic, energy healer and empath.

After profoundly transformational experiences back in 2010 of being in higher states of consciousness and seeing beyond her reality, she caught glimpses of her Higher Self and saw through the illusion of pain and suffering. She opened up to infinite human potential, realised that magic is all around us permanently and so committed to becoming a true vibrational catalyst in order to help raise the vibration of the planet and empower others on their ascension path.

Combining all the tools picked up along the way, including energy healing and coaching, she now helps people in a unique way to deeply connect with their Higher Self in order to create a life of unconditional love, flow and inner peace.

Connect with Karin online karinmarieeke.com
For Quantum-Touch: https://bit.ly/KarinQTwebsite
YouTube : Youtube.com/channel/UCUDxmdykJRujOh2e79Bsqwg
Facebook : Facebook.com/groups/985205621653689
Instagram : Instagram.com/karin_eke/

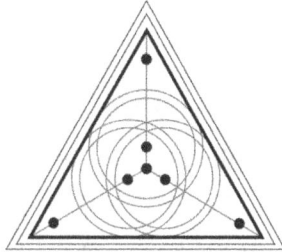

Part 4
Integration of Mind, Body and Soul

Now that you have a good sense from our authors of how, no matter the external circumstances, it was the internal shift that made the difference in the healing process, it is time for our last section of stories. The authors in this section are all here to share with you their individual journeys to integrating the parts of themselves that were left out in the cold, and returning to their original, whole state. These stories really embody the message of this book — body and mind cannot be separated, and we need to love and trust our whole selves.

Whether you think of yourself as having a soul, a spirit, or an essence by any other name, it all amounts to the same idea. We each came here with a purpose that is as individual as our fingerprints. Our soul's health is just as important to our healing as our mental or physical health, and so purpose cannot be left out of the equation. And sometimes, the soul and our connection to beings beyond our awareness, can save us when we aren't able to save ourselves.

As you will hear from Judith, a brilliant pioneer in EEG neurofeedback and meditation, the purpose she uncovered is to teach the methodology that freed her from feeling trapped and helped her find her way in the world. For our other authors in this section, it is a similar theme but each with a unique story of aligning with either their soul's purpose, or freeing their mind from turmoil, leading to healing their body. The word 'freeing' is important to pay attention to. As you will see in Shelley's story, she found learning to surrender a big part of her healing process and the spiritual assignment she is now committed to sharing with the world. She has since dedicated her life to bringing forth a methodology for surrender and functional medicine coaching. Delia, a gifted energy healing mentor and life reinvention strategist, saw that facing her emotions allowed her to tune into the messages from her soul, which led to deep healing. And Vidya, a talented IT product manager, decided to go on an investigative **journey** of soulwork to get to the root **cause** of her debilitating sciatica and back pain. Her ongoing practice of meditation and yoga keep her thriving and active today.

May these stories inspire you to look beyond your illness or pain for wisdom from the soul that renews your vitality.

When All Else Fails, Surrender

by Shelley B. Thomas, JD, NBC-HWC

Removing the cape

My heart dropped to my stomach when he looked at me and said, "You're only as happy as your saddest child." How could he have known? Everyone else at work thought I was Teflon. One of my favorite managers affectionately referred to me as her "barracuda" since I had mastered the ability to influence doctors' treatment protocols in ways that very few reps had achieved. I had great success as a drug representative; winning countless awards, lavish trips, lucrative bonuses, and all the accoutrements of building multi-billion dollar product franchises.

But today was different. Until now, I had been masking my grief and hiding my insecurities under a veil of perfectionism; always proving I had it all together. Now that I was exposed, ironically I felt comforted. I was suffering and that was my truth. Although it felt akin to working in my birthday suit, it was indescribably liberating. No longer was I compelled to perpetuate this shallow facade that I had mastered. Now the healing could begin.

My earliest memory of feeling vulnerable occurred when my father moved to Texas while I was in grade school. Dad was a Renaissance Man, the most intelligent man I knew. I couldn't have asked for a better father and friend. However, each time Daddy left for Texas on Sunday evening, I felt an indescribable well of abandonment, a bottomless pit of suffering. No matter how many times he returned home on the weekends, it felt as if I'd never see him again as he drove out of sight; leaving me standing tearfully in our picture window, watching until his tail lights faded into the distance.

A child never fully heals from feeling abandoned. In my eyes, my dad was perfect. I always looked forward to spending exciting summers boating on the lake, attending the theater, or simply visiting my friends in Texas, the best part of all. Unfortunately, however, his absence created a perpetual vulnerability in my soul that became a magnet for additional trauma which multiplied throughout my life.[1] It was an ever-present cloud over an otherwise perfect childhood.

As a child, I never questioned why I had frequent bouts of stomach discomfort, or why we kept a bottle of Maalox on my nightstand. Nobody I knew went to therapy back then, or spoke casually about depression like my friends and I do today. In those days, African American women were expected to be hyper-resilient; always donning a virtual Superwoman cape and appearing flawless like a tower of strength. For as long as I can remember, I believed that I was a descendent of royalty. In my mind, I'd inherited the fortitude of my forefathers who had survived the middle passage. So why did I feel so unbelievably fragile with all of the opportunities I had been given?

As my mask began to crack, the depth of my exhaustion peeked beyond the veil of my warm smile and obliging demeanor. It took every ounce of determination that I could muster to juggle the demands of a competitive career, community leadership roles and single parenthood to a twice exceptional child.[2] Less than one year after moving into our scenic hilltop home, my son transitioned from participating in the nation's top program for gifted children to showing signs of high functioning autism and grave developmental regression. At night I buried my tears so deeply that I began to believe my own tale of relentless superpower.

---

[1]Centers for Disease Control and Prevention. Publications by health outcome: Adverse childhood experiences (ACE) study. Atlanta, GA: Centers for Disease Control and Prevention; 2012.

[2]https://peakgifted2e.com/what-is-twice-exceptional-2e/

I felt incredibly guilty for causing his head injury when he was a toddler by failing to secure a child proof gate at the top of a steep flight of stairs, while momentarily distracted for what seemed like milliseconds. I remain haunted by images of him plunging down those stairs, less than three feet from my grip, and watching his head hit the concrete floor below. Once again, I buried this trauma deep in the graveyard of my memories.

When the student is ready, the teacher will appear

~ Lao Tzu

Instead of enjoying high school socials, playing sports or excelling in his pre-engineering program, much of Nick's time was spent with doctors seeking answers to this nightmare that kept me awake more nights than I care to remember. If I wasn't working, I was taking him to appointments or tutors to keep him afloat. At night I escaped to my bed where I began hibernating with countless hours of mind-numbing television to recover from the idiopathic illnesses that surfaced after moving into our new home.

Life had become a nightmare. I was entrenched in fights with our local school district to provide adequate accommodations. It was as if I was the only person concerned about Nick's wellbeing. Much like any teenager, Nick grew tired of feeling different from his peers. Every effort to "fix him" was met with unwavering resistance that threatened his emotional wellbeing and college admissions. I knew we were no longer working towards a common goal. For the first time ever, I listened to my son's insistence that I should redirect my energy towards saving myself; and I surrendered.

Exhausted from a slew of ailments ranging from adrenal dysfunction to unresolved asthma, I was burnt out and no longer inspired to save myself or anyone else. My health began declining more than ten years before my accident. I was never able to achieve any meaningful relief with the medication I was prescribed. All of my concerns were summarily dismissed or trivialized at best, despite having reached the point where it took a minor miracle just to work each day.

One beautiful spring afternoon, life was interrupted. I was en route to visit one of my favorite customers who practiced rural medicine in a remote community nearly four hours away. I looked forward to our weighty conversations and efforts to solve the world's problems. He jokingly referred to me as a Type AAA personality who always demanded his undivided attention. This day began no differently from any other until an hour into the drive I began experiencing grave fatigue like never before. This wasn't the feeling of staying up late the night before, which I hadn't. Instead, I became alarmed by red flags that warned me to pull onto the shoulder of the highway. But within seconds, I had blacked out. I traveled at least twenty additional miles while unconscious, without fatally injuring myself or anyone else. I don't understand how I maneuvered so well and was able to safely exit the highway before hitting a traffic sign in the intersection of two state highways. Had I traveled another five hundred feet beyond the exit ramp, it's likely that I would've driven off an overpass, killing myself and many others on the highway that day. I was surrounded by angels.

I walked away from the accident without a scratch. Though somewhat concerned about my job, I was grateful to be alive despite feeling like I was dying inside. Aware of the risks I took while driving long distances for work each day, I became more determined to find the cause of my failing health.

Shortly thereafter, I was led to Aunna, a brilliant, young, compassionate physician who permitted me to tell my story and share the wounds which had festered inside for far too long. Unlike many conventional doctors, she didn't rush me or belittle my instincts. Something about her was different. So I trusted Aunna to help me understand why I felt as if I was dying.

With one single visit and extensive lab reports, I learned that my body no longer had the capacity to recover from any major stress or illness. My telomeres told a story that conventional labs couldn't explain. Examining my health on a cellular level revealed excessive cancer cells, autoimmune disease and several other conditions triggered by my history of trauma, a stressful lifestyle and inadequate self care. I finally knew why I felt like I'd been dying a slow painful death. I wasn't familiar with Functional Medicine, but now I had access to state-of-the-art labs, a gifted physician and progressive protocols for reclaiming my health.

Reclaiming My Power

I was given a second chance. For the next year or so, I worked obsessively to overcome my suffering and reverse the diseases that stole my health. Some days it felt impossible to eat another meal of nuts, seeds, and organic foods that tasted nothing like my favorite dishes. My relationship with food changed dramatically from being the highlight of every social gathering, to becoming medicine and the key to my survival.

My lifestyle was complicated. Like many, my diet wasn't the only cause of my suffering. As I continued to unravel the causes of my failing health, I learned that every trauma and my Type AAA personality (i.e., perfectionism) had each contributed to an excessive toxic load of volcanic proportions.

The Functional Medicine protocols exceeded my expectations. Not only was I able to restore my health and reverse my autoimmune disease, but I felt ten years younger. However, I knew there were additional changes I needed to make before I was entirely healed. Aunna warned, "Your job is going to kill you." I knew she was right, but I didn't know how to start over.

I found a gifted coach who taught me the art of resilience. With her coaching, I discovered that I had given all of my power to doctors, employers and anyone who seemingly possessed the keys to my authentic happiness. At that very moment, I vowed to reinvent my life! I gave myself one year to become healthy before turning fifty. With that charge, I tested my home for toxins, employed spiritual warfare and otherwise commanded the Universe to help me manifest my best life. I discovered toxic mold in our home, the reason for my son's cognitive impairment. After remediating the mold, I then systematically treated every root cause of my illnesses.

I was like Rambo! Before turning 50, I was promoted at work and had attracted a romantic love interest who made me feel at least ten additional years younger. I celebrated my birthday with a lavish trip to South Africa where my son and I inhaled the serenity of the sunrise safaris and high tea at five. I connected with nature in ways I never imagined possible. I had discovered my fountain of youth and the ability to manifest my best life.

My new life exceeded my expectations. It seemed surreal! Sometimes I questioned if life could get any better. For the next year, my beau and I experienced the joy, play and wonder that somehow escaped me in adulthood. Whether experimenting with international recipes or exploring quantum physics, everyday felt as if I was running through a field of lilac and jasmine.

With my disability in the rear view mirror, I felt invincible! I was starting to believe that I was immune to stress, then life happened. A year into our relationship, my significant other developed bipolar disorder, my brother was in an accident leaving him in a coma with a traumatic brain injury, my mother was diagnosed with an aggressive form of cancer, in the same week an aunt died, and two close friends passed away unexpectedly from breast cancer. The Universe was clearly testing my resilience.

To my surprise, I remained as cool as a cucumber. Armed with sophisticated functional medicine protocols, training in Ayurveda and progressive spiritual practices, I responded to these stressors with poise and grace. It had been three years since my last disability and I thought I had passed the ultimate test of my resilience. I was prepared to accept my divine assignment to restore balance in the world and teach others what I had learned.

Secrets Revealed

Just one month shy of the launch of my new health coaching business, the impossible happened. The toxic mold returned and my immune system crashed from the excessive stress of the past year. Like before, my toxic load exceeded my capacity to overcome disease, and I became incapacitated, barely able to walk, leave bed, digest food, or think clearly. This time I wondered whether I now had cancer. My immune system was too compromised for Traditional Chinese Medicine and my specialist estimated that it'd take at least ten years and stem cell replacement to fully detoxify my body.

There was no magic elixir this time. I felt defeated. So once again, I surrendered. I abandoned my dream home and walked away from every possession we owned to save my family. I tried every available protocol, without an ounce of relief. Years earlier, my son experienced a miraculous shift in his health, academics and overall happiness when I surrendered my efforts to fix a seemingly impossible situation. Now that I had exhausted all available options for myself, I knew I needed to surrender again.

For the next year, I immersed myself in Mind Body Medicine, the same techniques used to help orphans recover from the traumatic effects of war. Each time I applied a new technique, my body made measurable improvements. Initially I was preoccupied with severe pain and discomfort. Recognizing that any misstep could trigger another relapse, I cautiously embraced this opportun new

By the time I had completed the advanced training, I was pain free at last! The connection between my willingness to surrender and my ultimate healing was unmistakable. I learned that when you pause to find meaning in your suffering, you're more likely to achieve deeper healing and find a greater purpose for your being.[3]

For several months thereafter, I searched my soul to better understand my suffering. My assignment to teach the importance of living with balance was undeniable; and it wasn't lost upon me that I had been given the opportunity to learn from some of the greatest healers of our time. Yet I remained confused about this recurring illness that seemed determined to devastate my life. I knew there had to be an explanation.

That's when my spiritual mentor introduced me to Callings by Gregg Levoy. It confirmed my belief that illness was simply my soul's way of communicating a deeper message about my personal calling or assignment. Like the cosmic two by four that caused my near fatal accident years earlier, the subsequent ailments existed not because any protocol failed, but rather because I hadn't learned the greater lesson for my suffering. Levoy taught, "If we medicate our symptoms away or get them 'fixed' by the doctor, hoping to return to our lives and pick up where we left off without missing a beat, then we've missed the point of the pain. Fortunately and unfortunately, though, the opportunity to grow will come around again."

Eureka! I finally understood why so many people with complex illnesses often experience recurring symptoms or successive ailments long after treating the original disease. Success lies not only in healing the physical body, as I achieved with the reversal of my

---

[3]Dr. Bernie Siegel, "Love, Medicine and Miracles".

autoimmune disease, but also in healing the mind and spirit, by surrendering to learn the lessons buried deep in our souls. Just as we each have a unique set of genes, each person's journey for healing requires a personalized blueprint. There's no single algorithm for reversing disease. You are not your diagnosis.

For me, the deeper healing began with acknowledging the history of trauma that I'd numbed with Maalox, perfectionism and suppressing memories too painful to recall. Neuroplasticity rewired my brain. Functional Medicine healed my body. Ayurveda personalized my care and reclaiming my power accelerated resilience. But nothing was more powerful than surrendering to the Universe for spiritual attunement and detoxification. I now have every tool I needed to heal my body and work towards manifesting my very best life.

About the Author

Shelley Thomas is a retired Pharmaceutical Executive, an Attorney and Board Certified Health and Wellness Coach. She is the founder of My Healthcare Partner, a Lifestyle Medicine practice which seeks to eradicate needless suffering in the world. Shelley is an avid student of personal development, human consciousness and a meditator with a passion for manifesting health, wealth and actualizing your best life through the art of surrender.

For more information about reversing disease with evidence based lifestyle modification practices targeting the root cause of disease, connect with Shelley at www.myhealthcarepartner.net.

The Healing Mirror

by Judith Pennington

What I love most about life is its mirror-like nature, in which we see who we are and what we want to be. As we grow older, we look deeper into our mirrors, systematically removing obstacles to our hopes and dreams. Sometimes we are not aware of walking the path of destiny, but when we meet it, we look back and see a lifetime of synchronicities that led us to where we were meant to be.

I started out as a curious, observant journalist in search of personal healing and found an inner portal to universal healing. For the past fifteen years, I have used a unique electroencephalograph, the Mind Mirror, to guide people all over the world to the healing wisdom of the subconscious soul: the inner mirror that is truly the fairest one of all.

Healing did not come to me easily, as I seem to have arrived in this world with a strong-willed, skeptical mind that wars with my intuitive spirit. As a child, I sensed a sacred presence in nature and the candlelit sanctuary of my Catholic church, where the glowing beauty of stained glass, fragrant incense, and the soaring harmonies of the choir lifted me into mystical union and a peaceful love for all of life. I rejected my spirit as a teenager, but at age twenty-two, when I was diagnosed with a serious medical condition, an extraordinary event changed the course of my life.

I was driving my red Karmann Ghia to my doctor's office for a follow-up visit when I heard myself sending up a prayer: "If there is a God, please don't let anything happen to me. There's no one else to take care of my little girl." Suddenly, a cold chill swept through me then burst into waves of warm light that exploded into joy and bliss. I threw my head back and surrendered to the radiant white light, weeping in gratitude for this invisible force that knew and loved me. Words cascaded into my mind: *You are loved without end and have never been alone, nor will you ever be. There is no death. This is what it feels like to die. There is nothing to fear.*

That spontaneous illumination dissolved a large tumor on my left ovary, and without realizing it, I set out on a quest to find out what had healed me. *Had it come from inside or outside of me? And could it happen again?* My questions went unanswered for fifteen years, until I asked once more for help and was guided to the science of spirituality and powerful ways to heal and be healed.

By age thirty-seven, I was a busy freelance writer, the director of a peace and justice group, and the single mother of two daughters. I was successful professionally, but my body was wrecked. A skating fall onto my tailbone and two car crashes had left me with neck and back injuries so painful that I dragged one leg behind the other. I could not afford to pay for healing, so life lined it up for me through a series of story assignments that required me to experience the holistic therapies that were making their way to my hometown of Baton Rouge, the capital city of Louisiana.

Hot yoga, a sensory deprivation tank, hypnosis, biofeedback, and massage in a heated swimming pool relaxed my tense, rigid body, and as the fog of pain began to lift, I was assigned to write about several well-known psychics who opened my mind to my spirit. In one large class on psychometry, I plucked a woman's name out of a basket and saw a detailed image of purple flowers that turned out to be the design on her blouse, which was hidden under her jacket. Then I investigated a California psychic who traced on a map of Louisiana the location of two murderers driving to a swamp to dump the dead body of their victim. State police followed the psychic's lead and apprehended the killers.

Several of the psychics I interviewed did readings for me which were so accurate that my walls came tumbling down. Intuition is of the spirit, they told me, and I felt the truth of this. In late 1987, I finished writing a personality profile that I knew would open the hearts and minds of readers, and as I prowled around my bedroom at 2 a.m., in that twilight between asleep and awake, I felt an inner impulse that said, "Sit down, pick up pen and paper, and record what you hear."

I met in my "writings" a wise, loving presence that called me to a goodness much greater than my own. In the years ahead, their universal laws always reflected the challenges in my life and inspired me to choose the path of love. Transcendent perspectives flowed into my opening heart and clarified my mind and life. I did not know where the guidance came from, but I deeply trusted my inner voice, especially when its predictions of coming events proved to be true.

I was learning to love myself, but only because my writings said that self-love is the "carrier of the Light": the light that heals and transforms us in the quiet of the mind and the love flowing in the heart. "The Light" was identified as the energetic power within beauty, love, goodness, and joy. Soon, my inner voice predicted, I would understand it as a tangible force.

A few days after that prediction, a newspaper assigned me to write about a former NASA physicist speaking at a local healing center. His explanation of the electromagnetic wave spectrum of light jolted through me like a lightning bolt. Suddenly everything made sense! The reality we process with our physical senses in the bandwidth of visible light is only a sliver of the existing frequencies. I realized in a flash of insight that the photonic light spoken of in my writings is real, and it literally carries the energy of light into existence within and all around us.

It was clear to me that my spiritual illumination at age twenty-two occurred through resonance with a higher vibration of light. I knew and had felt that light as pure love. Some give it a face and call it God.

Each epiphany loosened the stranglehold of my ego and lifted me higher and higher up into my spirit. The impetus was always the guidance of my psychic soul; the result was always deep personal healing.

In 1989 one of my writings said that I would soon have an opportunity to be purified in Medjugorje, Yugoslavia. And indeed, in that spiritual power point I did release heavy burdens of guilt and shame. As my spirit soared, higher levels of wisdom and love flowed into my writings. One day, I walked to the top of a tall, craggy mountain without any back pain at all.

From that point on, I lived in wonder. The predictions of my inner voice synchronized with external reality, and in that state of flow I felt loved and supported as never before. Even my chronic back pain was alleviated after a 1993 writing said that I would soon learn to meditate and find great healing in it. A series of unlikely coincidences led me to an Edgar Cayce study group, which I participated in weekly for ten years.

In the first meeting, I opened the introductory chapter on meditation in the *A Search for God* study group text and found directions on how to meditate and a description of God as the energy of light, which agreed with everything my writings had been teaching me for the previous seven years.

The Cayce style of meditation, dating back to the late nineteenth century, came naturally to me, as my writings turned out to have been a form of meditation. I sat in silence each day for an hour, and that luminous field of love and joy did indeed instill a lasting sense of peace in my mind, emotions, and spirit. Cayce, the "sleeping prophet" and father of holistic healing in America, recommended chiropractic treatments, an eighty percent alkaline diet, and the application of castor oil packs, all of which reduced the inflammation in my spine and decreased my pain levels by half.

By 1999, I was eager to follow my writings' twelve years of predictions that I would write a book sharing their universal wisdom. I spent a month on retreat in Virginia Beach selecting them and writing a short narrative suggested by an editor for the book, titled *The Voice of the Soul*. But upon completing the narrative, I realized that I had no objective proof of my claims that meditation and meditative writing awaken our psychic abilities, lucid dreams, synchronicity, and healing.

I asked inwardly for proof, and a clear, sharp vision of "Common Boundary" magazine led me to its cover story on Anna Wise, titled "The Brainwaves of Healing." Wise was mapping and training brainwaves—the electrical activities of consciousness—on a unique electroencephalograph (EEG) called the Mind Mirror. She used it to usher meditators to the ideal Awakened Mind brainwave pattern, a symphonic orchestration of frequencies which awaken the mind to the wisdom, light, peace, and guidance of what she called the "essential being" and I call the soul.

The brainwave science of Anna Wise and her teacher, English biophysicist and Mind Mirror inventor C. Maxwell Cade, proves scientifically that meditation awakens all of the abilities I had claimed in my book. I realized that my meditative writings had developed my own brainwaves to awaken my mind, step by step, over the previous twelve years. You could have bowled me over with a feather.

In 2005, my writings urged me to study with Wise. Specific courses of action had never been suggested before, so I overcame my argumentative ego, followed the guidance, and studied for a year with Anna toward certification as an Awakened Mind Consciousness

Trainer. I used the Mind Mirror to guide people to the inner healer, and it proved to be an infallible fast-track to personal integration. In deep, profound meditation, it is easy and painless to clear outworn, unhelpful attitudes, thoughts, and behaviors embedded in the subconscious mind, where healing must occur for it to last.

Over the past fifteen years I have led thousands of people into the Awakened Mind brainwave pattern for self-discovery, healing, and transformation. Not once has a client, student, or subject been unable to make that soul connection. Reuniting with the true self always enhances creativity, insight, intuition, empathy, and spirituality.

After Anna passed away in 2010, I founded the Institute for the Awakened Mind, traveled the world to certify practitioners, and co-developed a Mind Mirror that processes super-fast gamma frequencies that synchronize the brain and accelerate learning, intuition, healing, and spiritual transformation within superconscious levels of awareness.

Time and again, I have seen high-frequency gamma affect people in wondrous ways, especially in large-scale research programs at The Monroe Institute. It is there that I've led a team of Mind Mirror practitioners over the past three years to monitor the brainwaves of people engaged in remote viewing (psychic perception) and out-of-body travel. Some people heal, some attain mystical union. Most of them psychically view or travel out of body to identify the hidden target photo or object with an incredibly high rate of precision and success.

I have seen and experienced great wonders on the Mind Mirror, and all of it is living proof of the infinite intelligence within us and our ability to attune to different frequencies and dimensions to accomplish the seemingly impossible.

It is my great joy to conduct these studies on non-local awareness, as well as my ongoing research on healers and healing. Such is the definition of one's life work: it benefits us and at the same time serves our communities and the world.

In 2019, I traveled to the Rhine Research Center at Duke University to study the brainwaves of a famous healer, Edd Edwards, who transmitted high-amplitude gamma waves while we were both hooked up to the Mind Mirror during a ten-minute healing session. The last piece of scientific proof I needed for my theories on light fell into place when a biophoton device measured increases in the coherent light Edd emitted and we shared. I was completely free of pain for six weeks: healed by the light of compassion and love, just as my writings had always said and the science that followed them repeatedly proved.

Then, a few months later, while I was in San Diego to monitor the opening and closing brainwaves of thirty-five people attending a Life Visioning Retreat conducted by Dr. Dawson Church, my deeply held longing for another spiritual illumination was fulfilled. While my hand was on the shoulder of a man seated at the center of a healing circle and other people connected with us in a closed energy loop, I prayed for his healing and waves of bliss cascaded through my atoms and cells. I wept with joy for the return of that healing light. When I returned home, I had ten times more healing gamma waves than I'd had before, and it was integrated with my super-sensitive body, just as I had needed and asked.

Such are the promises of gamma frequencies and their attunement to the higher vibrations of the electromagnetic wave spectrum of light.

With and without gamma, I have seen Awakened Mind training help countless people clear psychic pain and get a new lease on life. Lost souls find themselves in a world of hope. Widows reunite with their departed husbands. Elderly men weep with gratitude when they are finally able to say goodbye to their long-dead parents. All of this occurs in the mirror of the soul, beyond the boundaries of time and space.

I am inexpressibly thankful for every moment of my life, including the injuries which set me on a path to healing, that my soul might guide others to theirs. Since these last two healings, my pain levels are less than twenty percent of what they were to begin with. When I live in the light of my spirit, as I have done while writing this story, there is no pain at all. I know that complete healing will come when the time is right. Keeping faith with that draws me ever closer to it.

I believe that we are always healing and transforming, as these are the laws of nature and life. But I also feel that humankind is on the verge of a quantum leap in evolution as people turn inward and open to their hearts and souls. It does not matter what the catalyst is, only that we believe in the possibility of healing, ask for it, and trust in the mirror of the soul to guide us to the light of love.

All the light we need is within and all around us. When we look inside its radiance, what we see is our true nature of pure, perfect Light.

About The Author

Judith Pennington, the author of two books and seven guided meditation albums, lives among the cornfields and blue hills above Bethlehem, Pennsylvania. She invites readers to learn more about the brainwaves of consciousness on her website at www.InstitutefortheAwakenedMind.com and to experience the transformative array of mind-awakening meditations available at www.MindMirrorPortal.com.

Facing my emotions

by Delia Sanchez

It was November 2017 and a cold, sunny Saturday morning in the beautiful Lake District in the UK. As I was waking up, I realised that I was in one of my favourite places on earth. I took a long, deep breath feeling so grateful for that moment and for everything that was waiting for me. It was the first day of a wonderful one week break. As usual when I was there, I knew that my stress was going to disappear. The place seemed to have a magical power to turn off the sense of urgency and necessity while turning on the necessary and oft-forgotten reminder to slow down, be present and be mindful.

A trip to the Lake District had always been a joyful, planned getaway with the simple goal of recharging. I'd always book the same room so that rest was ensured.

Grasmere is situated in a charming village nestled at the foot of some spectacular fells. It even has its own lake. I return because the place ticks all the boxes for me — lush green surroundings, lakes, streams, delicious food, hikes and runs in the hills, silence and beautiful dark skies. So yes, that morning I woke up in my idea of paradise.

I got up and went across to the balcony to listen to the clear stream that ran nearby. I could hear the ducks and other birds as well as the gentle sound of sheep in the distance. I spent a few minutes there just taking it all in. 'I love this place,' I thought.

As I turned away from the window, my reflection in the mirror caught my eye. I couldn't help but notice my mouth. I'd developed an eczema-like rash around the edges of my lips making it look like I had a double mouth with undefined edges. In my eyes, it was ugly and impossible to hide. I immediately forgot my beautiful surroundings and came back to my reality where I felt unattractive and even ugly.

My self-esteem was at rock-bottom and I just wanted to hide away from social situations where I felt that my mouth would be on display. When I was outside, I would cover my mouth with my hands and ask friends not to look at me. Things were not good.

The rash was uncomfortable and itchy at times. I had online consultations with a few doctors and they had each given their vague explanations of what they thought it might be. They would suggest some creams or lotions for me to put on it but none of them had worked for long. As a pharmacist, I am convinced that using any type of medication should be a last resort. I never used any medicine unless it was absolutely necessary. However, I was desperate. I wanted a solution fast. After talking with the third doctor and getting a third prescription, this time for the inevitable corticosteroid cream, I decided to give up.

I used the cream while knowing that I was just treating the symptoms and not the cause. I would use it to a point where the rash was no longer uncomfortable, then I'd stop for a few days before starting again. From a treatment point of view, I knew that this was not the right thing to do.

I remember constantly being in victim mode. Why me? When will it end? What if it never goes away? These questions were on my mind the whole time. I felt irritated, frustrated and angry.

During this time I was working in e-commerce. I wasn't happy with my position and felt like I'd wasted my time and money. I noticed that no matter how hard I worked, I never moved up. The work was monotonous and felt like a heavy chore. Many days I felt unhappy with my progress.

The first time I noticed eczema was after a family discussion with my brother and my dad. It was after I'd organised a family trip then received a call from my brother who'd said that he was no longer going with us. While I understood and had actually been expecting this to happen, I was still disappointed. To make it worse, my dad had then called and cancelled the trip.

It may sound silly to you, but I'd always dreamed of having a family trip together. All my friends at school had them. I'd been so excited and had arranged everything. That's why when my dad phoned to cancel, my heart had broken. It had taken me back to my childhood summer holidays when everyone's families had travelled together except for ours. I hadn't been able to stop crying for about a week after this. That was when the eczema had appeared.

I am sure that by now you've already connected a few pieces from my story. So, let's go back to that beautiful hotel room. It was another day of feeling sorry for myself, feeling miserable about everything and in addition I was feeling guilty about it. After all, I was in one of my treasured places and just couldn't enjoy it. Suddenly I received a message from a friend with a reminder about a self-help energy healing course that he'd mentioned to me about 2 weeks before. It was due to start the following day and it was going to be online (so no excuses!). He hadn't only invited me to join, but he'd said, "I will do it with you."

Let me tell you more about this extra special friend. He knew what I was facing, he knew how disappointed and frustrated I was about everything. He didn't say much (he is a man of few words). He just invited me and because he knew me so well, I didn't have other options but to accept the invitation. This was because one year before that, he'd convinced me to go on a 10 day silent meditation retreat. At first I'd been reluctant to go but it had been one of the best things I'd ever done in my life. So, this second invitation meant a lot.

The following day, I was there and ready with my notebook, pen and my favourite ginger lemon tea. The course began and as the minutes passed by, I found that I was totally engrossed in what the teacher was saying. It had all made total sense to me. The more she spoke, the more excited I became. "Why have I never thought about this before?" I asked myself. She explained the challenges we face in our lives in a way I hadn't thought of before. I wrote down a lot during that course and experienced an uncountable number of 'aha' moments. My mind was on fire trying to absorb as much information as possible.

Eventually, she'd stopped talking and had asked us all to stand up. She moved onto the practical part of the course and as we started with the exercise, I felt an instant connection to it. It was so easy to feel, notice and experience what she was asking us to do. I felt like I'd surrendered and let my body or whatever force was acting on me just speak for me.

Suddenly, I had the most intense feeling I've ever had. My heart was beating fast with excitement. I closed my eyes and saw myself in a space with no walls, slowly turning around in it. I didn't realise it at the time, but it was a space of infinite possibilities. In that moment of excitement, eagerness, agitation and energy, I said to myself, "I will never stop doing this!" The words hit me like thunder, strongly and deeply. I felt this powerful intention being imprinted on every cell of my body. And to think that this was just day one out of five in the course!

The following four days were magical. I loved every part of them — the reflections and the exercises. I was a hundred percent present. As the course was coming to an end I already knew that I wanted to continue learning about the technique. So I signed up to what became the most intense, difficult yet rewarding 10 months of my life to master the technique.

The eczema was still there but my attention wasn't on it as constantly as it had been before. After the trip, I booked a consultation with a therapist who specialised in various energy techniques, including the one I'd learned in the course. These sessions investigated the root cause of my problem such as checking my emotions, issues and challenges and connecting it all together.

After a few sessions, the eczema was still there, however, I was looking at it from a different point of view. It was like my physical body was showing me my emotional issues. These issues were stamped into my face, so they could not be hidden away but had to be faced! Since then, there hasn't been a day that I haven't use these techniques.

The course helped me to face all the demons and monsters inside me (I didn't know that I had so many!) It had been extremely difficult to go back in time and remember things, situations and people that I had just wanted to forget about. However, the deeper I went, the deeper the work had been and the lighter I felt after it.

I remember creating a list of every negative situation I'd ever been in and a list of every person I'd ever met for whom I'd had a negative feeling. I looked over every family member (alive or dead). One of my main issues was that I'd suppressed the pain of my mother's death and never grieved properly. After ten years, I couldn't even look at her picture. Happily, I finally had the courage to do so. It was a liberating experience that was full of love, as it is meant to be.

After a few months, the eczema began to disappear. This motivated me to continue. Actually, by then I had many reasons to continue working. I was feeling energised and had a positive mindset. This started to open doors and bring opportunities my way. I even went on a business trip to Bangkok — something that I never would have imagined doing before. I also landed my first big e-commerce client who later became my main client. There were yearly trips to the magical island of Bali, Indonesia included in the contract.

Today, I can tell you that I'm so grateful for the eczema I had. All my issues were literally written on my face. This caused me to dig deep inside with the single purpose of understanding and discovering the best version of myself. I understand now that our physical bodies are constantly talking to us and when we don't listen, they will make themselves heard another way. I know now that no matter how painful and difficult a situation is, it's better to deal with it right then and there. I've stopped hiding things under the carpet but rather face them in the moment. I feel calm and have learned to trust. I decide what to feel, how to feel and I recognise that I am the only one responsible for what I feel. Most importantly, I keep mastering myself and learning about who I am. I understand the power of a thought and the intensity of a positive vibration. Today, I am consciously choosing how I want to live my life.

Now, as an energy trained mentor and therapist, I feel one hundred percent myself. I feel complete. I have found my soul career and I work to show others what is available and completely possible to whoever is willing to face their dark side and finally encounter the bright side. I help them find the most real and beautiful side of themselves. I connect with those who feel the eagerness to walk that extra mile and achieve the once-thought unachievable dream. Today I am focused on keeping soul, mind and body as they should always be — together.

Today I look at the mirror and love what I see! Do you?

About the Author

Delia C. O. Sanchez is a pharmacist, biochemist and has a master's degree in pharmacology. After spending many days in silent meditation retreats, she developed a passion for energy healing. After successfully overcoming several career changes, today Delia is an Energy Healing Mentor, Meta Health Practitioner, Archetype Coach, Soul Career Finder and Life Reinvention Strategist.

As of today she has empowered many clients around the world, including UK TV celebrities, on finding their own connection to their real and most beautiful version of themselves.

As healer and teacher, she is committed to her mission which is a #consciousreinvention movement in partnership with bestselling author, international TEDx speaker and media personality, Dr Andrea Pennington. Together they empower many others to find the real version of themselves and consciously reinvent their lives.

Connect with Delia on social media:
www.instagram.com/deliacosanchez
https://www.instagram.com/the_reinvention_club

Sciatica Relief, The Natural Way

by Vidya Mahabeleswar

Jan 3, 2004

I remember it like it was yesterday. We had just moved into our new home, the first home we had ever owned. New Year's Eve had just passed. I'd had an amazing holiday that included a road trip down from San Francisco to LA and Vegas, friends visiting from all over the country and an absolutely wild NYE party. My visitors had all left, and the morning of the 3rd was when I was due to return to work.

It was dawn and as I opened my eyes, I saw the sun rising through our bedroom window and the glistening rays making their way to warm up all that they could touch. The next thing I recall is that I simply couldn't move. I tried lifting myself up, but in vain. It was as though my spine was stuck to my bed. Tears started rolling from my eyes due to excruciating pain in my back. I turned over to my right and saw that my husband was still fast asleep. I decided not to wake him up, and since my bed was a low platform bed, I rolled off the bed on my left side, still in a lying position. Badly needing to use the bathroom, I started to crawl using my elbows on the smooth hardwood floor. Inch by inch, every move I made sent chilling pain into my back and legs. Those few feet felt like the longest distance to travel and many thoughts were going through my mind.

I somehow pulled myself up once I made it to the bathroom. Holding on to any support I could—the door, the walls—I relieved my bladder, which at that point seemed non-existent. The fact that I couldn't use the restroom as I normally would made my mind spiral. Would I be able to stand up at all? Would this pain go away, did I need to call for an emergency? Would I spend the rest of my life in a wheelchair? How did this happen and why me?

I had no answers, just a lot of questions, and a lot of pain. I had always loved travel, the outdoors and driving to exotic places. I pictured myself in my 20s, spending my life in a wheelchair and this made me cry harder. I screamed for help and my husband came and got me, and took me back to lie on my bed. I couldn't go to work that day and I started making plans for what I needed to do next. The events that followed changed my life in ways I could not possibly have imagined.

I called my doctor's office for an appointment. I also called my sister-in-law, who is a Physical Therapist, to get some advice. The X-rays and MRIs showed that two discs in my lower back were herniated (an abnormal bulge or breaking open of a spinal disc). This was the cause of the sciatic pain that ran through to my left leg. The doctors suggested spine surgery, stating that 10% of cases show full recovery.

I took swift treatments including massages, spine stretches and exercises to strengthen my lower back. I still had to take pills, several days worth of muscle relaxants, and a high dose of painkillers. These helped somewhat and meant that I could get back to work after a few days. But did the pain go away? No.

The quest for a sustainable solution

I used to drive a Nissan Sentra stick shift car that I had fondly bought during my graduate school days. Each time I hit the clutch with my left foot, shooting pain went down my legs. I ended up donating that car. I couldn't go back to practising tennis with my husband. There was a group of friends that played volleyball on weekends and I couldn't imagine ever playing again as the doctors said that any activity involving jumping would make my pain worse. So there were days when I just sat by the courts and watched others play.

I relied on painkillers such as Motrin, Ibuprofen so that I could do some activities. Then came a turning point. It was winter and we went to Lake Tahoe, which is a range of mountains with ski resorts. I was new to skiing and had taken a few lessons, however, for those with sciatic pain, skiing is another sport that can aggravate the pain. I held back and didn't attempt it on this trip. I sat watching all the skiers speed down the snowy slopes, waving their arms with joy. I so wished one of them was me. When we returned home, I took to doing more research on the ways that people manage pain. It started opening my mind up to a myriad of possibilities! I was excited, hopeful and determined.

I tried to understand what sciatica was. It is one of the most common, yet misunderstood, types of pain. As many as 40% of people will get it during their life, and it becomes more frequent as you age—according to Google. The sciatic nerve is the longest nerve in the human body, and the pain I was feeling was caused by a compressed (or pinched) nerve. Many health websites suggested that there are pain management experts, who again would prescribe more drugs to manage pain. I wasn't going to settle for this. Something told me there was a better way. There are three approaches that led to a healing journey for me—and I'd like to share them with you now.

The first step

First, it was as though some divine intervention helped me to find a yoga studio close to home. It was in the corner of an intersection, a small space. Upon stepping up to the reception desk by the front door, the scent of essential oils, the warm, cozy decor and soft sounds took me over. I enrolled for a prenatal class as I had just learnt I was pregnant. My instructor Colleen introduced herself. She originally came to yoga with a chronic back injury and had discovered its profound healing benefits for herself. Colleen's story and her restorative style of teaching rekindled in me the hope that I'd make strides towards being pain free.

Everything about this yoga class started to feel like this was meant to be. The main hall of the studio was rectangular, about 25 feet deep and would fit around 12-15 people. The walls were painted mustard yellow and orange shades on the windows made it cozier. At the start of our classes, the subtle aroma of scented candles coupled with soothing chants meant my senses would drift away to a distant place and my pain would momentarily vanish. So every Saturday morning up until my 9th month of pregnancy, I showed up on my mat at the yoga studio. Mainly because of this, I glided through putting on 40 plus pounds and recovered from labor without having to take pain medications for my sciatica.

Yoga then became a part of my daily routine, whether it was starting my day with 12 surya namaskars (sun salutations), or following a YouTube routine with a few different yoga teachers at the end of the day. As my child started growing, my pain came back with a bang— I suspect this was from all the weight lifting, and having to juggle work, home and a child.

Deeper discovery of alternative approaches

This time I did something different. I didn't go back to my regular doctor. Instead, there was a second approach that helped me— Acupuncture. A friend's wife who had been a dancer had also experienced sciatica. She told me about an acupuncturist from China that she went to. Her back pain went away to the point that she could dance again. I was petrified of needles, yes even for a mother who's been through childbirth, needles are still scary! But I decided to give it a try.

I met Doctor Helen, who has been an acupuncturist for over 20 years. Her steely smile and confidence reassured me when I lay there on the table, facing down and completely trusting someone to shoot needles into my body. Sometimes, she put needles in the back of my ear and at times on my pinky toe. I didn't quite understand how it would work, but in just a few sessions my back loosened up and I felt amazing. I also shed the extra pounds I had gained due to pregnancy. Doctor Helen had said this might happen. Over time, I reduced my trips to Helen as I moved far away from her clinic. I supplemented by continuing to do yoga practices.

By this point, several years had passed since I had that first episode of being unable to move, but something was still unsettling in me. I didn't feel I understood the root cause of body pain. The more I read about the cause of back pain, inflammation and the western approach to diagnosing and treating pain, the more I could see that it didn't make sense to me for the longer term. I managed my pain and would say I knew how to deal with it, however I wanted to build more strength. I wanted to be able to drive long distances and to play certain sports and not fear that I would get stuck and become unable to move.

Then, out of the blue, in the fall of 2015, something miraculous happened. I say out of the blue because I had not ever tried meditation. I was drawn to attending a meditation workshop by yogi and mystic, Sadhguru.

My life's silver bullet

This is what led to my third approach for dealing with my pain—Meditation. Meditation or Dhyana (in Sanskrit) is a limb of yoga, according to Patanjali's Yoga Sutra, which is a classical yoga text.

If you'd asked me a few years ago, I would have told you that I couldn't sit still to meditate because I've always been very restless. I was always busy doing this, that and the other, with a huge social life. I was traveling, performing in dances, hosting theme parties, shuttling kids to their activities, working, the list would go on. What

I didn't know was that I would be swept up and rebirthed once I was initiated to a powerful meditative practice.

The two day workshop had a prerequisite of seven courses to be completed. I stayed up late after the family was asleep and completed the courses feverishly, in the nick of time. I showed up at 7am on a Saturday for the workshop. Among the hundreds of people that were part of this, I found some who were drawn to it for the very same reason as me, that burning question—what is the source of pain? In some cases the pain was physical, in other cases it involved mental or emotional suffering. I was convinced that this was going to be the silver bullet.

Those two days flew by as if they were just a few seconds, but towards the end of it I felt a new life come to me. I've since attended a few retreats and learned other meditative practices that are able to cure illnesses that to western medicine were apparently incurable.

Looking back to see how I got here

Now when I look back, I understand that I owe my success to going down the holistic route rather than allopathy. This road was not all that easy. I could write a book with many chapters on how these practices went at times. My little boy would be playing with his toy cars, but as soon as he saw me on my yoga mat, he would climb up on my back, while I was in a downward dog pose. There was the day when I sat to meditate and right then, my husband started looking all over the house for tax papers, opening every drawer, every cabinet. Another day, I hid in a quiet spot to meditate, and my daughter turned on the blender to make a smoothie that she suddenly craved.

These incidents are fun memories and they make me chuckle at my persistence to not give up. Because I kid you not, sciatica is like an evil twin—anytime outward stress increases, so it intensifies its presence. They also say the brain amplifies pain substantially as a consequence of stress, anxiety, and fear. So by taking pain medications, the symptoms are reduced but the root cause still remains. Once you start taking the pills route, your medicine cabinet just keeps expanding.

Of the many learnings I've had on this journey, many are deep and surreal. The stillness brings about radiance, the quieting of the mind brings about vitality, focus brings an awareness of the highest priority. There have been many triumphs along the way, telling me that what I'm doing makes sense. And this is why I want to share my story so that many more can benefit from it.

No turning back from the holistic way

Remember when I watched people play volleyball and I sat outside wondering whether my back would spasm if I joined in? I recently played for four hours (with a lunch break in between). I followed up in the evening with gentle yoga stretches. On a road trip last year, I drove a huge Chevy Suburban for four straight hours and hiked the next day for six straight hours in the Zion Narrows. I woke up earlier than normal to practise my meditation.

I've not only started skiing with my family, but I've also advanced from the bunny slopes to blue level runs, and I'm hoping to get to some harder blue slopes in the future. I once had the image in my mind of me sitting in a wheelchair. This has now been replaced by pictures of me on the top of peaks. Amidst all this, over time the connections I have made with people who follow holistic ways of living has been nothing but fascinating. I feel the sense of deep knowing and yet yearn for more, to know of alternate ways of healing. I have experienced in mystical ways how the different energies play out in the universe. I have in the past kept this journey to myself. However, through this medium I now believe that in some corner of the world someone may be going through the same struggle, and that they may benefit as I did.

After all the years of finding these ways of dealing with pain, I have just one question to ask anyone who tells me that they have been diagnosed with sciatica, and that they are on medications. You perhaps can guess it: Have you tried yoga and meditation? There may be skeptics at first, however, the more stories are shared, the more holistic treatments are asked for and are considered by the medical profession.

About the Author

Vidya Mahabaleswar uses storytelling extensively in her professional life as a technology product leader. Her desire to reach more people who can benefit from sharing her triumph in her health quest led her to tell her story as a co-author in Holistic Healing. With over a decade and half of research, including experiments adapting several holistic approaches to lifestyle and diet, Vidya has gained successful outcomes that have proven to be sustainable.

Vidya is a regular practitioner of traditional Yoga, meditation and also an avid promoter of plant based food consumption. She lives in the San Francisco Bay area with her family and enjoys gardening, biking, hiking and travel. Her latest spirit of inquiry is observing life through the lens of her teenage daughter.

Vidya is interested in connections that aspire to bring a holistic and natural lifestyle to a wider audience.

Connect with Vidya on LinkedIn:
www.linkedin.com/in/vidya-mahabaleswar-6057847

Conclusion

By now, I hope you are thinking about your own health and healing from a more holistic perspective.

By now you know that we cannot separate the mind from the body, or heal one without the other. And here in our 3-dimensional reality we also need to make space for our soul, spirit, essence, or however you choose to describe it. Just because we can see it does not mean that we aren't influenced by it.

Personally, I believe that we all came here to live our lives on this planet with an individual purpose as our Authentic Self. Typically, it is when we find ourselves out of alignment with that purpose that unhappiness and discontent sets in. From there, discontent over time turns into disease, as we struggle in an endless battle of push and pull between our soul's purpose and what society is telling us to do. And when we try to conform to other's expectations or deny our own true desires, we lose the connection to our healing power.

Personally, not living in alignment with my soul's purpose manifested as depression and anxiety. First, as a young medical student working nearly 100 hour weeks in the hospital, I had stopped making time for my first love, music. I was too busy being a student doctor to notice that my soul was gradually getting sicker — until I finally fell into a deep, black pit of despair.

Many of us experience something similar. I followed my father's wishes and studied medicine, as he had instilled in me the belief that music was a hobby and not a profession. And while I did enjoy the nerdy aspects of medicine, and I've continued to work in and around the health field, I needed to incorporate more of my true self into my daily life, including into my work.

The battle between should and want

This battle between what we believe we should do with our lives, and what we want to do with our lives is a big one. But it's made even harder by the fact that our bodies and our minds are entering the adult world of societal pressure and responsibility, already damaged by childhood trauma that we haven't learned to process and heal.

If you find yourself wondering why you haven't moved on fully from your own childhood trauma, then please know that you are not alone, and it is not a failure on your part. We were never taught how to, and that is a failure of society, of the human race at large.

We all collectively need to bring healing holistically, and learning to acknowledge and process our pain into mainstream society. We need to give ourselves and each other permission to be the complex human beings that we are. It is no small feat, as I'm sure you can imagine. And we won't get there overnight. But I do feel that the world is gradually waking up.

With the global pandemic of 2020, so many people have been thrown off their well-trodden track that they were given by their parents or leaders. Instead of following instructions, people are being forced to reassess what life really means to them. We are all being called to investigate how spend our time and how we are damaging our health over the long term.

Although we are all hurting from the pandemic in the here and now, I do wonder if it will bring a silver lining. I wonder if this is the beginning of the end of this era, and perhaps a time of great change is coming. Perhaps we will all begin planning our lives based on our soul's purpose. And maybe we will even teach our children and grandchildren how to heal themselves from their trauma and pain — or avoid being wounded in the first place!

Conclusion

So I would like to leave you here with these reminders. You are here on planet Earth, reading this book. The fact that you are reading this book means that you are alive — your time on Earth is not yet done. You have life left to experience and to influence. So what might you do next? What do you need to heal first?

And when you heal, what might you choose to do that invokes your passion and your soul's purpose? Do you know what your purpose might be, or is there a voyage of discovery yet to be taken?

Please don't put this book down and let the ideas you have go. What happens next is entirely up to you. So will you take a step in a new direction?

Please visit the websites and social media accounts of each of our authors to connect more deeply with their work if you are so inspired. They are generous, compassionate souls who are committed to making the world a healthier, happier place.

You can download some of my guided meditations and other free resources from the authors to help you with your own personal healing journey at www.HolisticHealingBook.com. You can also watch video interviews with them there and on our YouTube channel.

We wish you a life full of vitality, purpose and peace.

Resources

If you would like to calculate your own ACE (Adverse Childhood Experiences) score, then visit the link below.
http://bit.ly/findyourACEquiz

The questions in the quiz are from the CDC-Kaiser Adverse Childhood Experiences (ACE) Study. The Centers for Disease Control and Prevention ACE Study uncovered a concerning link between childhood trauma and chronic diseases, plus social and emotional problems developed later in life. Much research has been inspired from this, and understanding your own ACEs can be a solid starting point to your own healing journey.

Watch interviews with the authors and download their free resources by visiting the book website:
www.HolisticHealingBook.com

About the Book's Creator

Dr. Andrea Pennington is an integrative physician, acupuncturist, meditation teacher, and international speaker who is on a mission to raise the level of consciousness and love on our planet. As a personal brand architect, media producer, and communications specialist, she leverages her 20+ years of experience in broadcast and digital media to proudly help healers, Light workers and coaches to bring their brilliance to the world through publishing and media production with Make Your Mark Global Media.

Dr. Andrea is also a bestselling author, international TEDx speaker and documentary filmmaker. For nearly two decades, she has shared her empowering insights on vitality and resilience on the *Oprah Winfrey Show*, the *Dr. Oz Show*, iTV *This Morning*, CNN, the *Today Show*, LUXE-TV, Thrive Global and HuffingtonPost and as a news anchor for Discovery Health Channel. She also produced a four-part documentary series and DVD entitled *Simple Steps to a Balanced Natural Pregnancy*.

Dr. Andrea has appeared in many print publications including *Essence, Ebony, Newsweek, The Sun, Red, Top Santé* and *Stylist*. She has also written or contributed to 13 books. She is the Founder of the #RealSelfLove Movement and hosts the *Conscious Love, Conscious Evolution* and *Conscious Branding* podcasts. As Founder of In8Vitality she blends her 'nerdy' mix of medical science, positive psychology, and mindfulness meditation to empower us all to show up authentically, love passionately, and live with vitality.

Visit Dr. Andrea online at:
AndreaPennington.com
RealSelf.Love
MakeYourMarkGlobal.com
In8Vitality.com

Get Social!
facebook.com/DrAndreaPennington
twitter.com/drandrea
linkedin.com/in/andreapennington
instagram.com/drandreapennington

Other Books Published by Make Your Mark Global

Manifesting Love
Created and Compiled by Andrea Pennington

The Top 10 Traits of Highly Resilient People
Created and Compiled by Andrea Pennington

The Real Self Love Handbook: A Proven 5-step Process to Liberate
Your Authentic Self, Build Resilience and Live an Epic Life
by Andrea Pennington

The Ultimate Self-help Book: How to Be Happy, Confident & Stress
Free, Change Your Life with Law of Attraction & Energy Healing
by Yvette Taylor

Magic and Miracles
Created and Compiled by Andrea Pennington

Life After Trauma
Created and Compiled by Andrea Pennington

The Magical Unfolding *by Helen Rebello*

The Orgasm Prescription for Women
by Andrea Pennington

Time to Rise
Created and Compiled by Andrea Pennington

The Book on Quantum Leaps for Leaders: The Practical Guide to
Becoming a More Efficient and Effective Leader from the Inside Out
by Bitta. R. Wiese

Holistic Healing

Turning Points
Compiled and Edited by Andrea Pennington

How to Liberate and Love Your Authentic Self
by Andrea Pennington

The Top 10 Traits of Highly Resilient People (Summary)
by Andrea Pennington

Daily Compassion Meditation: 21 Guided Meditations,
Quotes and Images to Inspire Love, Joy and Peace

by Andrea Pennington

Eat to Live: Protect Your Body + Brain + Beauty with Food
by Andrea Pennington

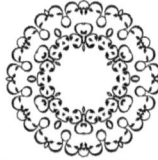

MAKE YOUR MARK GLOBAL

Get Published
Share Your Message with the World

Make Your Mark Global is a branding, marketing and media agency based in the USA and French Riviera. We offer publishing, content development, and promotional services to heart-based, conscious authors who wish to have a lasting impact through the sharing and distribution of their transformative message. We also help authors build a strong online media presence and platform for greater visibility and provide speaker training.

If you'd like help writing, publishing, or promoting your book, or if you'd like to co-author a collaborative book, visit us online or call for a free consultation.

Visit www.MakeYourMarkGlobal.com

Call us at +1 (707) 776-6310 or

send an email to Andrea@MakeYourMarkGlobal.com

www.ingramcontent.com/pod-product-compliance
Lightning Source LLC
Chambersburg PA
CBHW050729030426
42336CB00012B/1485